THE FIT SWIMMER

120 WORKOUTS & TRAINING TIPS

THE FIT SWIMMER

120 WORKOUTS
& TRAINING TIPS

MARIANNE BREMS

Contemporary Books, Inc.
Chicago

Library of Congress Cataloging in Publication Data

Brems, Marianne.
   The fit swimmer, 120 workouts and training tips.

   Bibliography: p.
   1. Swimming—Training.   2. Physical fitness.
I. Title.
GV837.7.B74   1984   797.2'1   84-4355
ISBN 0-8092-5454-9

Published by Contemporary Books, Inc.
180 North Michigan Avenue, Chicago, Illinois 60601
Manufactured in the United States of America
Library of Congress Catalog Card Number: 84-4355
International Standard Book Number: 0-8092-5454-9

Published simultaneously in Canada by Beaverbooks, Ltd.
195 Allstate Parkway, Valleywood Business Park
Markham, Ontario L3R 4T8 Canada

To all those I've trained with, taught, and coached, from whom I've learned so much

CONTENTS

FOREWORD

Each day as I walk into the pool, I like to have a plan for my workout. I am constantly looking for new approaches which will do at least one of the following, and possibly all three:

1. give me a change from normal routine
2. make me a faster swimmer
3. challenge me to work harder

In her book, Marianne Brems has addressed these needs in an informative and entertaining way. Rooted in a firm foundation of scientific training principles, she provides her readers with a wide choice of workouts which will assist those at any swimming level to accomplish such goals.

Marianne's excellent skill as a Masters swimmer, a coach, and a knowledgeable writer serve to make this book a valuable resource. It is a welcome addition to every swimmer's library from the beginning fitness swimmer to the national record holder.

James E. Counsilman
Swimming Coach
Indiana University

ACKNOWLEDGMENTS

I am sincerely grateful to Dr. James E. Counsilman, not only for taking time from his hectic summer schedule to write the Foreword for this book, but also for being a genuine supporter of my project. I hold his respect in particularly high esteem because, reputable and celebrated as he is as a coach, he hasn't been afraid to get his own feet wet and swim with the rest of us.

I also wish to thank Harald Johnson for throwing the files of photographs at *Swim Swim* magazine wide open to me. A large number of additional photographs were, on short notice, expertly taken by Dave Gray and processed by Bob Cossins.

I am further indebted to Gina Gatto for her patience in producing the manuscript, for help with selecting photos, and for faith and encouragement all along the way.

To Lynn Zito I owe thanks for providing me with pertinent comments concerning her early impressions of open water swimming, as well as for suggestions for improving the manuscript.

1

INTRODUCTION

The main purpose of this book is to promote the idea that swimming can provide a path to lifetime personal fitness. Beyond that goal, I have specifically addressed those questions that most often arise concerning training sessions. Such questions include: Where do I start? How much time should I spend swimming? How hard should I push myself? How can I get the most out of my time in the water?

In considering the answers to these questions, it is clear that the greatest benefit comes from a consistent and persistent program of training. So it is with the understanding that no satisfactory substitute exists for time and effort spent training on a regular basis that I have created the workouts in this book.

In addition, I have borne in mind the idea that this training should be fun. After all, to my way of thinking, winning in swimming must go beyond the feeling of touching the wall first at the end of a race to the sensation of maintaining youth and vigor year after year. And you're certainly not going to swim for a lifetime, no matter how good it is for your body, if your workouts become drudgery.

As an aid to helping you avoid such a predicament, this book tells you how to determine your swimming level and choose your

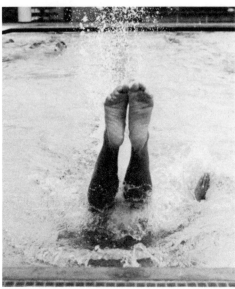

Getting your feet wet!

Photo by Harald Johnson

workouts accordingly so that, on the one hand, they don't deplete your energy for other important activities in your life and on the other, you do challenge yourself and elevate your heart rate to an appropriate level for a suitable length of time.

This book is intended for those who want to swim for fitness as well as for those who want to prepare for pool or open water competition. It provides appropriate workouts for swimmers who have never trained before and know only the most basic stroke technique as well as for the highly trained athlete. In short, the book furnishes the novice and the record holder with a comprehensive collection of challenging yet stimulating workouts designed with the latest training concepts in mind for the purpose of keeping the reader interested in swimming.

HOW TO GET THE MOST OUT OF THIS BOOK

At the basic level, the way to get the most out of this book is to *do* the workouts regularly. And there's no substitute for starting *now*.

Early in your training, however, you will want to make some decisions. In general, you must decide what you will give in exchange for an increase in your energy level and a heightened sense of well-being. Then decide, more specifically, what level of conditioning you want to attain and when you want to reach it. This implies knowing from where you are starting, which you can determine from examining Chapters 3, 4, and 5. Also, look closely at your overall weekly activity schedule and decide how many days a week you want to swim. Then make each workout a high priority in the day's program. After making these basic decisions, you may also wish to think about any particular aspects of your training that you want to emphasize, such as building endurance or increasing your leg strength.

Familiarize yourself, if necessary, with the training terms in the Glossary so that you will understand the workout notations as you plan your practice sessions in the water. Also, make sure you are acquainted with the training equipment if you intend to use it. When reviewing the checklists for proper stroke mechanics, have a coach or experienced instructor examine your strokes, if possible, and help you evaluate your skills in regard to the various points on the list.

When doing the workouts themselves, it is not necessary to follow the order in which they appear in the book. In fact, I would suggest that you pick and choose from among the workouts included, depending on your needs and desires. An exception might be the first 12 workouts in Chapter 3, "Beginning Workouts," which progressively build the total distance per workout from ¼ mile to 1 mile. And even if you find yourself using beginning workouts, don't be afraid to choose periodically a workout from the intermediate (Chapter 4) or advanced (Chapter 5) category—both for variety and to spread your wings. You can always adjust the yardage of the workout by the method suggested in the following section. By the same token, if you are in the intermediate or advanced category, you can always choose a beginning workout and increase the yardage and the number of individual sets you swim.

HOW TO INCREASE OR DECREASE THE YARDAGE OF A WORKOUT

Since age and level of ability, as well as the time for and interest in swimming that you create for yourself, vary so greatly, study the following procedure so that you can customize almost any workout to your particular needs.

In general, to reduce or increase the yardage of an individual workout, if the distance is short change the number of repeat swims.

Example:

Reduced Amount	Suggested Amount (Yards)	Increased Amount
6 × 50	12 × 50	20 × 50

In this example, if the swimmer were not advanced enough to do 12 50-yard swims, he or she could reduce the number of 50-yard swims to six. The more advanced swimmer, on the other hand, could increase the yardage by doing 20 50-yard swims.

If, on the other hand, the distance is long, alter the distance, but keep the number of swims the same.

Example:

Reduced Amount	Suggested Amount (Yards)	Increased Amount
3 × 200	3 × 300	3 × 400

In this example, instead of the suggested three 300-yard swims, the swimmer could swim either three 200-yard swims or three 400-yard swims.

Within the framework of a complete workout, the changes would appear as follows:*

———————— SAMPLE WORKOUT ————————

Distance	Stroke	Time
1 × 300	Free	Warm-up
6 × 100	Free	On 2:15
1 × 300	Pull: free	
12 × 50	Fly, back, or breast	On 1:10
2 × 150	Kick: fly, back, or breast	
6 × 25	Free	On :45
	3 breaths per 25 yards	
1 × 200	Free	Swim-down
2,450 yards total		

*Back = Backstroke, Breast = Breaststroke, Fly = Butterfly, and Free = Freestyle

This sample workout can be customized for the less advanced swimmer (Reduced Workout) and for the more advanced swimmer (Increased Workout) as follows:

Reduced Workout	Suggested Workout (Yards)	Increased Workout
1 × 200	1 × 300	1 × 400
3 × 100	6 × 100	9 × 100
1 × 200	1 × 300	1 × 400
6 × 50	12 × 50	18 × 50
2 × 100	2 × 150	2 × 200
4 × 25	6 × 25	8 × 25
1 × 100	1 × 200	1 × 200
1,400 yards total	2,450 yards total	3,400 yards total

2

DEFINING YOUR LEVEL OF SWIMMING SKILL AND SETTING GOALS

I have always found hitting a target you can't see to be excessively difficult. You're much more likely to get where you want to go if you know where you are as well as where you want to end up.

YOU ARE HERE

The most detailed and accurate map on the face of the earth is of no value to helping you reach your destination unless you know where you are starting from. I'm reminded of a large wall directory of the type often found in sprawling, multi-level shopping centers with the words "You are here" inscribed in bold letters at just the appropriate point.

Of course, when dealing with something as intangible as your physical condition, a "You are here" label is more difficult to position—and is difficult because your condition can change quite rapidly with only a slight alteration in your activity. Before setting fitness goals, you must know where you are now. Your heart rate, both at rest and during aerobic exercise, can tell you quite a bit about where you currently stand.

6

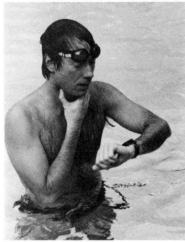

Photo by Harald Johnson

Measuring heart rate

Resting Heart Rate

To measure your resting heart rate, place your fingertips on your carotid artery (on the right or left side of your throat) before rising from bed in the morning and count the number of heart beats in 1 minute. This count will increase slightly with age, but will decrease (perhaps significantly) with exercise. In fact, adult swimmers that I've coached have often told me that the sense of well-being they gained from beginning a training program was accompanied by a drop in their resting heart rate after only a month or two. Depending upon your age and level of conditioning, a rate of 50–70 beats per minute indicates a better-than-average level of fitness.

If you regularly keep track of your resting heart rate, you will have the additional benefit of knowing when to take a day of easy swimming or a day off from swimming altogether. You should do this if your resting heart rate is elevated five or more beats per minute on any given morning.

For the purpose of goal-setting, your resting rate is of further use to you because you need this figure to determine a good exercise heart rate to aim for. To do this, you must also estimate your maximum heart rate (and I say "estimate" because the only accurate way to measure maximum heart rate is on a treadmill) by subtracting your age from 220, which is considered the theoretical maximum heart rate (reached at approximately age 10). For example, if you are 35 years old, your estimated maximum heart rate is 185 beats per minute (220 – 35 = 185).

Target Working Heart Rate

Once you have determined your maximum heart rate as well as your resting heart rate, you can find a safe and productive heart rate at which to do your swimming. According to DeVries,* this safe and productive heart rate during exercise is one that does not exceed approximately 60 percent of the difference between your resting and your maximum heart rates over and above your resting heart rate. So if, for example, your age is 35 and your resting heart rate is 60 beats per minutes, you would figure your target working heart rate as follows:

$$
\begin{array}{rl}
220 & \text{(your theoretical maximum heart rate)} \\
-\ 35 & \text{(your age)} \\
\hline
185 & \text{(your estimated maximum heart rate)} \\
-\ 60 & \text{(your resting heart rate)} \\
\hline
125 & \\
\times\ .60 & \\
\hline
75 & \text{(60 percent of the difference between your} \\
& \text{maximum and resting heart rates)} \\
+\ 60 & \text{(your resting heart rate)} \\
\hline
135 & \text{(your working heart rate during exercise—60} \\
& \text{percent of the difference between your resting} \\
& \text{and maximum heart rates over and above your} \\
& \text{resting heart rate)}
\end{array}
$$

This working heart rate is a good, safe level to stick with for the purpose of inducing fitness by swimming (about 12–20 minutes three times a week for a minimum standard). But be aware that, if you've been out of the water for years or have been virtually physically inactive, then the slightest exercise may initially set your heart racing, and I suggest practicing moderation until you can swim at the target heart rate. However, you are probably eager to accomplish something more from swimming than a minimum standard of fitness. If a higher level of conditioning or speed is what you are interested in and you're in reasonably good condition,

---

*Herbert A. DeVries, *Physiology of Exercise for Physical Education* (Philadelphia: W. B. Saunders Co., 1976), page 111.

swim portions of your training sessions at a rate that is equal to your resting heart rate plus *80 percent* of the difference between your resting and maximum heart rates. Plug this figure into the formula above, and you will get a working heart rate of 160 beats per minute.

Your Current Exercise Heart Rate

Now that you've done your paper work, it's time to find out what your actual working heart rate is so that you'll have an idea of how hard you are working when you swim, and where you stand. To measure your working heart rate, place your fingertips on your carotid artery *immediately* upon reaching the pool wall after a 10-minute swim and count the beats for 6 seconds, then multiply that number by 10 to determine the rate for 1 minute. For example, if your heart rate is 12 beats for 6 seconds, it would be 120 beats per minute. (The heart rate is counted for only 6 seconds both because taking your pulse for 60 seconds in the pool takes too long when you're dealing with short rest intervals, and because if you're well-trained, your heart rate will drop drastically in a minute, giving you an inaccurate working rate.)

So, once you know how to determine (through computation of your resting, target, and actual working heart rates) how hard you are working at present, you can decide what changes, if any, you want to make in your program. The rest of this chapter is designed to help you figure out where you want to go with your training.

SETTING YOUR GOALS

As mentioned earlier in this chapter, swimming 12–20 minutes three times a week at your target working heart rate will induce and maintain a so-called minimum level of fitness. But, "What if I want something more?" you ask. Quite simply, if you want more of a result, you need to exert more effort, and I suggest beginning by increasing your swimming time to, possibly, 30 minutes at a stretch.

If your first goal is to increase your stamina and the distance you can swim in one session, you may wish to follow the first 12 workouts in Chapter 3 for a 12-week period. When you finish, you should be able to swim a mile without stopping.

Aiming for Efficient Swimming

The basic principle we rely upon when we train is that if we overload our bodies' cardiovascular system, our bodies will grow stronger to meet the demand. Thus, we must realize that to go a great distance with the lowest possible heart rate is only part of the total goal of swimming for fitness. Otherwise, we would all try to creep along at a snail's pace—which even the most complacent, noncompetitive lap swimmers soon tire of.

While distance is not the total goal of your training, neither is the increased heart rate that must be reached and maintained in order to achieve cardiovascular fitness. If this were so, we would tear madly and without method down the pool, making every move as difficult as possible solely for the purpose of raising our heart rates.

So what is the unifying element that brings lap swimmers and competitors to common ground and eliminates the obvious extremes of both the snail's-pace and the helter-skelter swimming styles? The answer is simple: it is efficiency, which implies both greater speed and increased distance.

Just as a car is most fuel-efficient when it travels at a constant speed, keeping a consistent number of strokes per pool length when swimming long distances increases a swimmer's efficiency because it evens his pace and conserves his energy. Periodically during a workout, you should count the number of strokes you take per length. (If this count increases by more than a couple of strokes, you'll know that you are tiring, so your pace is slowing and your heart rate is probably increasing.) The good part is that the longer you train, the better conditioned you will become and the more consistent your pace will be.

As you get more conditioned or as your stroke mechanics improve (or if both occur), you become more efficient—that is, you can go faster and farther while expending no more energy than before. Thus, even if your technique didn't improve at all, you would be able to swim farther and faster as a result of the conditioning that the swimming alone has given you.

Once you can swim a mile without stopping, to continue gaining the same amount of training benefit from your workout, you will have to increase either your speed or your distance, or both. Of course, increasing your *speed* rather than your distance is far more time-efficient. Thus we have the concept of interval training.

Interval Training

The term interval training refers to a series of periods of submaximal exercise alternating with controlled, short rest periods. The purpose of interval training is to elevate the heart rate to levels higher than those that result from nonstop swimming and thus build cardiovascular fitness. The idea is that with brief rest periods in your workout (periods long enough to provide some rest but not long enough for your heart rate to drop significantly), you can push your swims harder and thereby gain a higher level of fitness. Interval training is used by serious lap swimmers and competitive swimmers, and all of the workouts in this book (other than the first 12) are built around this concept.

You'll probably find it more challenging to do your interval swims by leaving on a fixed departure time rather than taking a fixed amount of rest. For example, if you decide to do a set of five 100-yard swims, beginning each 100-yard swim every 2½ minutes (that is, 5 × 100 on 2:30), then you have an incentive to swim fast because you'll get more rest in between 100s (you can also read your time on the clock more easily); whereas if you know you'll get 20 seconds of rest no matter what speed you swim, some of the pressure to perform is gone. A rest "interval" can also exist in the form of a length or lengths of easy swimming interspersed between lengths of hard swimming, such as swimming 300 yards and doing every third length at an easier pace.

Normally, rest intervals should not be long enough to allow your heart rate to drop to a nonworking rate; nevertheless, rest intervals vary in length. As a general rule, interval training with short rest periods (that is, swimming time to resting time being a ratio of 6:1 or more) builds endurance more than speed. On the other hand, training with longer rest intervals builds speed more than endurance. In other words, when you do a set of 50-yard swims on :50 (and get only, say, 5 or 10 seconds of rest between 50s), you're increasing a different competency than when you do the same set of 50s on 1:20, which allows you to get about 30 seconds rest.

Interval training is useful whether you are training for distance, sprints, or open water events. If you wish to use interval training to prepare yourself for distances of 200 yards or more, use at least 50 percent of your training session to do distances ranging from the length of the event to 100 percent longer, using a 6:1 swim-to-rest ratio and making sure that your heart rate (that is, your pace) is as fast as you can make it without sacrificing consistent speed. The other 50 percent of your workout should include kicking, pulling, and some *repeat* swims (that is a series of swims of equal distance) that consist of shorter distances, longer rest periods, and a higher resulting heart rate.

If you want to prepare for sprint events (those less than 200 yards), increase the amount of swims consisting of shorter distances and longer rests and decrease your swim-to-rest ratio to 2:1 for 50s and 25s and to 3:1 for 100s, so that you can swim at nearly your maximum heart rate. Also practice some swimming with limited breathing, but keep up something of a distance base for conditioning purposes as well.

If you are using pool training to get ready for open water swimming, I would recommend doing as much as 75–80 percent distance swims, using distances from 50–150 percent of the race distance, depending upon how far you plan to swim in the open water. The remaining 20–25 percent of your program may be devoted to kicking, pulling, and interval swimming with a 6:1 work-to-rest ratio.

SETTING UP A TRAINING SCHEDULE—AND STICKING TO IT

Once you've given some thought to the particular type of swimming that interests you most, the next step is to decide how much time and effort you can put toward reaching your swimming goals and still be able to fulfill other important responsibilities in your life. Every aspect of your swimming routine must be geared to the long run and to sticking with it, since that's where the real benefit originates.

Swimming Organizations

Consider that, as you progress toward your goals, you may find it helpful and rewarding to have some immediate external gratification in addition to the less measurable, yet wonderful, changes going on with your physiology. Contact your local American Red Cross office and ask about the "Swim and Stay Fit" program, whereby you receive a certificate once your cumulative training mileage reaches 50 miles.

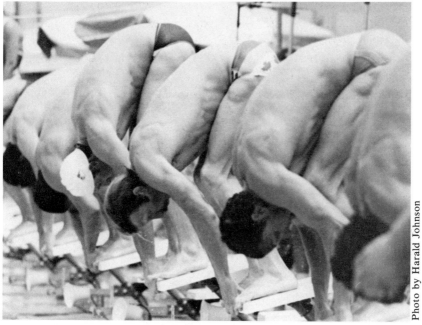

Photo by Harald Johnson

Competitive swim meets are held year-round on local, regional, and national levels.

Also, you may wish to try your wings at competition to measure your improvements in speed. Competitive swim meets on the local, regional, and national level are held year-round under the jurisdiction of United States Masters Swimming, Inc. Masters are adult swimmers 25 years of age and up who compete in age groups of 5-year increments such as 25–29, 30–34, and 35–39, up to 90 and over. In some regions there is also a 19–24 age group. Information concerning Masters as well as fitness swimming programs in your area can be obtained from *Swim Swim* magazine, 8461 Warner Drive, Culver City, California 90230.

Your Daily Schedule

Just as important as finding a swimming organization to connect with is taking a good, hard look at your own daily schedule. Then see how the lap swimming hours at the facility you will use coincide with the time you've allotted for swimming. Learn to view your time spent swimming as an investment in your own well-

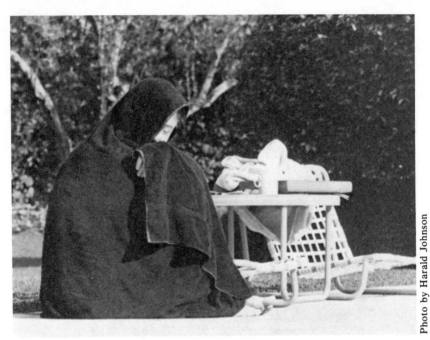

Photo by Harald Johnson

Be sure to stay warm after workouts.

being rather than as an additional load or intrusion into your day. I once heard motivational speaker and runner Zig Ziglar tell an audience that, for every minute of each day he spends running, he gains 3 minutes of productive time in return. I would suppose there is a point of diminishing return, but Ziglar said that he uses his exercise as a means of regaining energy after the exhaustion of delivering a speech.

So in that frame of mind, with swimming as a high priority in your life, decide how many days a week you want to swim. I would suggest a minimum of three and a maximum of six. Three days will keep you swimming regularly, and six will give you a day off for other things without feelings of guilt (in case you are so prone). And try to pick a number of sessions per week that you can *stick* with, because if you start missing a few sessions, it's usually easier to miss more. Besides, if you want to gain the benefits of swimming, clearly you must *swim*.

Next, decide how long you want to swim per session. Other than the initial adjustment period, if you wish to make use of the workouts in this book, swim 30–90 minutes per session, depending upon how competitive you wish to be, how much your workout takes out of you, and how many demands you have on your time. Again,

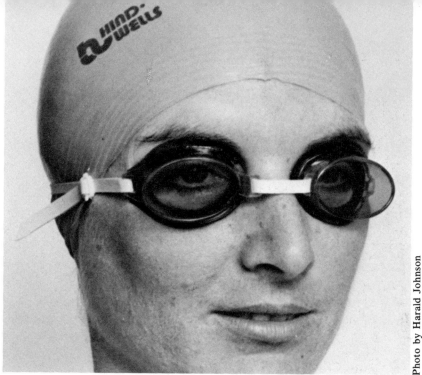

Photo by Harald Johnson

A swim cap will keep you warm, keep your hair out of your eyes, and protect your hair from those damaging pool chemicals. Goggles prevent eye irritation.

choose a program you can *stay* with consistently. Swimming for 90 minutes on three consecutive days and then not at all for a week is not as beneficial as swimming five times for 30 minutes during the same number of days—even though the total swimming time of the latter program is two hours less.

For relief and variety, you may wish to intersperse some days of easy swimming (rather than skip your swims altogether) with your days of more vigorous swimming.

Your attire during swimming should maximize comfort and practicality and minimize inconvenience. Wear a nylon or Lycra® swim suit (nylon lasts longer, but Lycra® feels sleek and is good for competition), since they create relatively little drag in the water and dry quickly out of the water. Most women find one-piece suits more comfortable than two-pieces. Use a cap to keep you warm, to keep your hair out of your face, and to keep your hair from becoming damaged by pool chemicals (not to keep your hair dry—it'll never work!) Also, most swimmers prefer to use goggles of the small plastic variety to prevent eye irritation both during and after swimming.

Now that you've given some thought to where you are and where you want to go, it's time to get your feet wet!

3
BEGINNING WORKOUTS

Once you've learned the basic swimming techniques of one or more strokes to the point that you can propel yourself for a couple of lengths of the pool, you're ready to begin a fitness program that can last you a lifetime.

So let's consider the standard for a minimum level of fitness— 12–20 minutes of exercise at a consistently elevated heart rate. With this in mind, you might wish to make your first short-range goal ¼ mile (which in the beginning will probably take you at least 12 minutes to complete) and your first long-range goal 1 mile.

But how, you may ask yourself, can you work up to those levels and beyond if, at present, you feel the need to stop and catch your breath far more frequently than every 12 minutes? The key is to use your heart rate as a guide (see Chapter 2 on checking your pulse) so that, on the one hand, you don't overdo your training and, on the other, you get an adequate workout.

As you begin your workouts, you will want to be aware of developing good breathing technique. Remember to exhale completely with your face in the water before rolling your head to one side to breathe. Avoid lifting your head or shoulders during inhalation, since this greatly increases the difficulty of breathing and tends to throw off the alignment of your stroke with each breath.

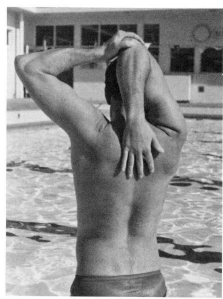

*Stretching helps you pre-
pare to start swimming.
Stretch your arms by reaching back and touching alter-
nate palms to the middle of
your back.*

Photo by Harald Johnson

Also, try to keep your strokes as long and relaxed as possible.
This will facilitate even pacing, which will conserve energy.
Concentrate on getting as much distance per stroke as you can
while keeping your kicks small and moderate, for kicking vigor-
ously requires a great deal of energy. In the beginning, take a
leisurely, I-have-plenty-of-time approach. After all, it's building

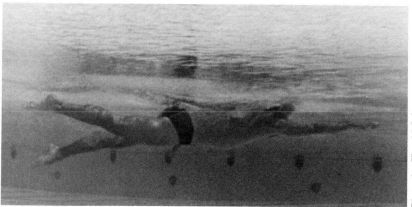

Photo by Harald Johnson

*To facilitate even pacing, keep strokes as long and
relaxed as possible.*

endurance, not speed, that's going to allow you to increase the amount you swim. If you're interested in speed, you can build that on top of an endurance base.

But above all, don't feel that you must have flawless aquatic technique before you can start building your level of fitness. All you really need—in addition to some very basic skills in stroke mechanics and the desire to improve—is a set of progressive workouts such as those in this chapter. If you're just beginning a program of regular training, or if you've been away from swimming for a long time, you may want to do the first 12 workouts in order. Do the workouts from three to five times each or for one week each, and thereby progress from sessions of 450 yards (approximately ¼ mile) to sessions of 1,800 yards (about 1 mile) in a period of twelve weeks.

WORKOUT 1 *

Distance	Stroke	Time
9 × 50	Free # 1–2: Concentrate on long strokes. # 3–4: Concentrate on proper breathing. # 5–6: Concentrate on small kicks. # 7–9: Concentrate on smooth, even pace.	After each 50, rest :45 or until heart rate drops to resting rate plus 40% of the difference between resting and maximum heart rates.

450 yards total (about ¼ mile)

EMPHASIS: Building endurance and proper technique in freestyle

If desired, advance to:

2 × 100	Free Concentrate on long strokes.	Rest after 100s as above.
5 × 50	Free # 1: Concentrate on proper breathing. # 2: Concentrate on small kicks. # 3–5: Concentate on smooth, even pace.	Rest after 50s as above.

450 yards total (about ¼ mile)

* Note that all the workouts in this book are geared to a 25-yard pool simply because this is the most common type of facility. If you train in a meter pool, multiply time intervals by 1.1 or add 5 seconds per 50 meters, 10 seconds per 100 meters, and so on.

─── WORKOUT 2 ───

Distance	Stroke	Time
3 × 75	Free	Rest :30 after each 75.
	Concentrate on even pace.	
75	Kick: free, with board*	
2 × 75	Free, progressive*	Rest :30 after each 75.
450	yards total (about ¼ mile)	

EMPHASIS: Building endurance; leg conditioning

If desired, advance to:

Distance	Stroke	Time
150	Free	
	Concentrate on even pace.	
100	Kick: free, with board	
2 × 100	Free, progressive	Rest :30 after each 100.
450	yards total (about ¼ mile)	

* See Glossary.

─── WORKOUT 3 ───

Distance	Stroke
150	Free
	Concentrate on long strokes.
75	Kick: free, with board
75	Pull: free, with pull buoy*
150	Free, progressive
450	yards total (about ¼ mile)

EMPHASIS: Building endurance; leg conditioning; arm strength

If desired, advance to:

Distance	Stroke
300	Free
	Concentrate on long strokes.
75	Kick: free, with board
75	Pull: free, with pull buoy
450	yards total (about ¼ mile)

* See Glossary.

──────── WORKOUT 4 ────────

Distance	Stroke
450	Free
	Every 3rd length, count your strokes per length. The more consistent the count, the more consistent your pace.

450 yards total (about ¼ mile)

EMPHASIS: Increasing your maximum nonstop distance; building a sense of even pace

──────── WORKOUT 5 ────────

Distance	Stroke	Time
450	Free, negative split*.	
150	Kick: free, with board*	Rest :30 at 50s as needed.

600 yards total

EMPHASIS: Increasing speed over a distance; leg conditioning

───────
* See Glossary.

──────── WORKOUT 6 ────────

Distance	Stroke
450	Free
	150:Concentrate on streamlining* off walls.
	150: Count strokes, holding number consistent.
	150: ripple stroke*
150	Kick: free, with board
150	Pull: free, with pull buoy and paddles*

750 yards total

EMPHASIS: Getting good distance off the walls; consistent pace; high elbows

───────
* See Glossary.

——————————— WORKOUT 7 ———————————

Distance	Stroke
450	Free
	Concentrate on relaxing.
150	Kick: choice of strokes, with board
150	Pull: choice of strokes, with pull buoy
	and paddles
150	Free
	Faster pace than in 450 above

900 yards total

EMPHASIS: Relaxing with freestyle; beginning conditioning in other strokes

——————————— WORKOUT 8 ———————————

Distance	Stroke	Time
2 × 450	Free	Rest 2:00.
	# 1: Concentrate on long strokes and high elbows on the recovery.*	
	# 2: Concentrate on even pace by counting your strokes every 6th length. Try to keep this number consistent.	

900 yards total (about ½ mile)

EMPHASIS: Increasing your maximum nonstop distance; lengthening stroke

* See Glossary.

——————————— WORKOUT 9 ———————————

Distance	Stroke
900	Free, negative split
150	Kick: choice of strokes, with board
150	Pull: choice of strokes, with pull buoy, paddles, and tube*
150	Choice of stroke (all the same stroke)

1,350 yards total (about ¾ mile)

EMPHASIS: Increasing speed over a distance; leg conditioning; building arm strength

* See Glossary.

―――――――――――――― **WORKOUT 10** ――――――――――――――

Distance	Stroke
900	Free
	300: Concentrate on streamlining off walls.
	300: Count strokes, holding number consistent.
	150: ripple*
	150: normal
450	150: choice of strokes
	150: free
	150: choice of strokes

1,350 yards total (about ¾ mile)

EMPHASIS: Improving push-offs from walls, even pacing; getting elbows up

―――――――――

* See Glossary.

―――――――――――――― **WORKOUT 11** ――――――――――――――

Distance	Stroke	Time
2 × 900	Free	Rest 2:00
	# 1: Stretch out, relax, extend off walls.	
	# 2: Maintain speed of # 1; keep strokes long.	

1,800 yards total (about 1 mile)

EMPHASIS: Gaining comfort with distance swimming while building endurance

―――――――――――――― **WORKOUT 12** ――――――――――――――

Distance	Stroke
1,800	Free
	450: Concentrate on getting into a comfortable pace.
	450: Concentrate on keeping kicks moderate.
	450: Concentrate on long strokes.
	450: Concentrate on being smooth and enjoying!

1,800 yards total (about 1 mile)

EMPHASIS: Testing your endurance

Once you've completed a mile without stopping, you easily have enough endurance and conditioning behind you to begin diversifying your training. By diversifying I mean that you may wish to begin concentrating in some specific areas such as: a particular stroke or strokes; sprint training to build speed; or long-distance swimming, which requires endurance. You may also want to spend extra time working on your personal areas of weakness in order to balance out your skills and conditioning.

As a means to accomplishing such objectives, the following workouts have been designed around the concept of interval training, which was discussed in Chapter 2. Interval training involves a series of submaximal bouts of exercise alternating with controlled, short rest periods for the purpose of building cardiovascular (heart and lungs) fitness.

─────────────── WORKOUT 13 ───────────────

Distance	Stroke	Time
200	Alternate 25 free and 25 choice of strokes.	Warm-up.
200	Free.	Breathe every 3 strokes (every 5 if possible).
20 × 25	# 1: free # 2–3: breast # 4–6: back # 7–10: fly # 11–14: free # 14–15: breast # 17–19: back # 20: fly	Rest :20 after each 25. (Substitute freestyle for strokes not yet learned.)
200	Your best stroke, broken*	Rest :10 at each 50.
8 × 25	Choice of strokes	On :45
200	Free	Swim-down

1,500 yards total

EMPHASIS: Breath control (useful in sprinting); individual medley (I.M.);*conditioning; leg strength

---

* See Glossary.

————————————— WORKOUT 14 —————————————

Distance	Stroke	Time
200	Choice of strokes	Warm-up.
3 x 150	50 back/50 breast/50 free.	On 3:15. Extend off walls.

3 x 150	Freestyle.
	    50 concentrate on stroke/50
	        medium speed/50 hard
		On 3:00

	Kick: free	2 x 2:15
		    :45 hard/ :15
		    moderate/ :30
		    hard/ :15
		    moderate/ :15
		    hard/ :15 moderate

4 x 25	# 1: fly # 2: back # 3: breast # 4: free	On 1:00. Dive.
200	Freestyle	Swim-down

1,400 yards plus 4:30 kick total
EMPHASIS: Improving last ¾ of individual medley; leg conditioning; sprinting

————————————— WORKOUT 15 —————————————

Distance	Stroke	Time

200	Free
	    50: long strokes
	    50: ripple
	    50: bilateral breathing
	    50: normal
		Warm-up

4 x 50	Pull: free, with pull buoy, paddles, and tube	On 1:15
3 x {	1 x 100 of back 2 x 50 of breast 4 x 25 of free Increase speed as distance decreases.	Rest :30 after 100. Rest :20 after each 50. Rest :10 after each 25.
4 x 50	Kick: choice of strokes	On 1:30
100	Free	Swim-down

1,600 yards total
EMPHASIS: Proper stroke technique and breathing in freestyle; sprint conditioning

──────────── **WORKOUT 16** ────────────

Distance	Stroke	Time
300	Free, bilateral breathing	Warm-up
	Alternate 25 back and 25 free.	4:00 continuous
	Kick, broken: Alternate 25 back and 25 free.	4:00; rest :10 at 50s.
	Alternate 25 breast and 25 free.	4:00; continuous
	Kick, broken: Alternate 25 breast and 25 free.	4:00 rest :10 at 50s.
6 × 25	Fly	On 1:00
6 × 25	Free, 2 breaths per length	On :45
200	Freestyle	Swim-down

800 yards, plus 16:00 swim/kick, total
EMPHASIS: Variety in general conditioning; speed

──────────── **WORKOUT 17** ────────────

Distance	Stroke	Time
400	Free: Swim each 100 progressively faster.	Warm-up
4 × 50	Free, fast	On 1:30
100	Choice of strokes, easy	
4 × 50	Choice of strokes, fast	On 1:45
100	Free	Swim-down

1,000 yards total
EMPHASIS: Speed in several strokes

──────────── **WORKOUT 18** ────────────

Distance	Stroke	Time
200	I.M., reverse order Alternate 25 kick (no board) and 25 swim of each stroke.	Warm-up
200	Back	On 1:30
4 × 50	Kick: back (no board; arms extended behind head)	
200	Breast	On 1:30
4 × 50	Kick: breast (no board; arms at sides)	
200	Free	On 1:15
4 × 50	Kick: free	
200	Free	

1,600 yards total
EMPHASIS: Leg strength, individual medley conditioning

———————— WORKOUT 19 ————————

Distance	Stroke	Time
300	Free	Warm-up
	100: kick	
	100: pull	
	100: swim	
6 × 50	Kick: choice of strokes	On 1:30
2 × { 100 75 50 25	Free Increase speed as distance decreases.	Rest :20 after each distance.
6 × 50	Pull: choice of strokes	On 1:10
100	Free	Swim-down

1,500 yards total

EMPHASIS: Building speed; leg and arm conditioning

———————— WORKOUT 20 ————————

Distance	Stroke	Time
300	Choice of strokes Alternate 50 kick and 50 swim.	Warm-up
4 × 50	Free Alternate 25 ripple and 25 long strokes.	On 1:30
4 × 50	Free Breathe every 5 strokes.	On 1:25
4 × 50	Free, descending*	On 1:20
8 × 25	Pull: choice of strokes, with pull buoy, paddles, and tube	On :50
8 × 25	Kick: choice of strokes	On :45
100	Free	Swim-down

1,400 yards total

EMPHASIS: Freestyle stroke work; breath control; arm and leg conditioning

---

* See Glossary.

WORKOUT 21

Distance	Stroke	Time
100	Free	Warm-up
75	Breast	
50	Back	
25	Fly	
100	Fly, broken	Rest :20 at 25s.
4 × 25	Kick: fly	On :45
100	Back	
4 × 25	Kick: back	On :45
100	Breast	
4 × 25	Kick: breast	On :45
100	Free	
4 × 25	Kick: free	On :40
8 × 50	Pull: free	On 1:15
100	Freestyle	Swim-down

1,550 yards total
EMPHASIS: General conditioning for all strokes

WORKOUT 22

Distance	Stroke	Time
300	Free 100: long strokes 100: ripple 100: normal	Warm-up
50s	Free Swim until you can't make the interval. Then swim 2 more 50s on last interval made.	Best 50-yard time plus :40 = 1st interval. Subtract :05 more on each subsequent interval.
3 × 100	Pull: choice of strokes	On 2:15
16 × 25	# 1–4: fly # 5–8: breast # 9–12: back # 13–16: free	On 1:00 On :55 On :50 On :45
6 × 50	Kick: choice of strokes	On 1:15
200	Free	Swim-down

1,500 yards plus 50s total
EMPHASIS: Even pace; arm and leg strength

─────────────── **WORKOUT 23** ───────────────

Distance	Stroke	Time

300	Free
	    100: long strokes
	    100: bilateral breathing
	    100: normal
		Warm-up

100 75 50 25	Pull: free with paddles and tube	Rest :10 per length after each distance.
100 75 50 25	Choice of strokes (all the same stroke)	Rest :10 per length after each distance.

100
75
50
25
	Free
	    Increase speed as distance
	    decreases.
		Rest :10 per length after
		each distance.

100 75 50 25	Kick: choice of strokes	Rest :10 per length after each distance
200	Freestyle	Swim-down

1,500 yards total

EMPHASIS: Arm and leg strength; general conditioning for sprints

─────────────── **WORKOUT 24** ───────────────

Distance	Stroke	Time

300	Free
	    100: kick
	    100: pull
	    100: swim
		Warm-up

6 × 50	Kick: free with fins	On 1:15
4 × 100	Free, descending	On 2:30
6 × 50	Pull: free, with paddles and tube	On 1:30
4 × 50	Free, descending	On 1:10
200	Free	Swim-down

1,700 yards total

EMPHASIS: Maintaining speed in freestyle; ankle flexibility; arm strength against
resistance

──── WORKOUT 25 ────

Distance	Stroke	Time
300	Free, bilateral breathing	Warm-up
100	Free	Rest :30.
75	25 breast/25 free/25 breast	Rest :30.
50	25 back/25 free	Rest :30.
25	Fly	Rest :30.
300	Pull: free Breathe every 6 strokes.	

800	Free
	    25 easy/ 25 hard/50 easy/50
	    hard/75 easy/75 hard/100 easy
	    /100 hard/75 easy/75 hard/50
	    easy/50 hard/25 easy/25 hard	

200	Free	Swim-down

1,850 yards total

EMPHASIS: Endurance

4

INTERMEDIATE WORKOUTS

The workouts in this chapter are designed for the swimmer who can complete approximately 1 mile of nonstop swimming and who has become accustomed to doing interval training using several different strokes. It is not necessary that you be able to perform every particular stroke, distance, or interval suggested here in order to benefit from the workout; in fact, extending yourself to greater limits is what working out is all about.

If, on the other hand, you can do the assignments in this section with little or no stress, I would suggest that you do whichever of the following seems most appropriate: (a) decrease the suggested rest time; (b) increase either the number of repeat swims in any given set of swims, or the distance of the swim(s); or (c) choose your workouts from Chapter 5, "Advanced Workouts."

As a test of your ability to do interval training at the level prescribed in this section, try doing 10 100-yard sets of freestyle with 20–30 seconds of rest in between. If you can manage this set and you have some skill in at least one or two other strokes, consider yourself at the intermediate level for the purpose of using this book. Don't, however, feel that this is binding; feel free to do workouts from any of the other sections. I recommend it for variety and because you may discover talents you didn't know you had. After all, you can always adjust the quantity of any workout by the method described in Chapter 1.

Heart rate can also be a good indicator of your level of conditioning. If you are a well-trained, intermediate-level swimmer, your heart rate during your 10 100-yard swims of freestyle will probably drop 40–60 beats per minute during a 30-second rest interval.

However, if your heart rate does not drop, don't use it as an excuse not to begin or continue with your training program. In my years of training adult swimmers, I think the statement that I've heard most often is some form of, "I can't do a quarter-mile. I've never done it before. Besides, I'd be much slower than everyone else." My response to this is: First, there's got to be a first time to be a fiftieth time; and, second, the amount of cardiovascular benefit that you derive from a particular activity or the fitness level you attain has nothing whatever to do with how much or how little or how fast someone *else* swims. Anyway, improvement is not only inevitable if you work at it; it's also exhilarating—which is perhaps the greatest reward of all.

────────WORKOUT 26*────────

Distance	Stroke	Time
3 × 150	Free # 1: pull # 2: kick # 3: swim	Warm-up Rest :20 after each 150.
100 2 × 50 4 × 25	Kick: choice of strokes (all the same stroke)	100 on 2:30 50s on 1:15 25s on :45
2 × { 200 2 × 100 4 × 50	# 1: free # 2: back or breast Increase speed as distance decreases.	Rest 1:00 after 200. Rest :45 after each 100. Rest :30 after each 50.
100 2 × 50 4 × 25	Pull: freestyle	100 on 2:00 50s on 1:00 25s on :30
200	Freestyle	Swim-down

2,450 yards total

EMPHASIS: General conditioning in several strokes

* Note that all the workouts in this book are geared to a 25-yard pool simply because this is the most common type of facility. If you train in a meter pool, multiply time intervals by 1.1 or add 5 seconds per 50 meters, 10 seconds per 100 meters, and so on.

——————————— WORKOUT 27 ———————————

Distance	Stroke	Time
400	Free, bilateral breathing	Warm-up
200	Kick: I.M. (no board with back)	
8 × 100	50 fly/50 back (twice)	On 2:30
	50 back/50 breast (twice)	
	50 breast/50 free (twice)	
	50 free/50 fly (twice)	
200	Pull: free, with pull buoy,	
	paddles, and tube	
16 × 25	Odd lengths: choice of strokes	On :40
	Even lengths: free, 1 breath	
	per length	
200	Free	Swim-down

2,200 yards total

EMPHASIS: Individual medley conditioning; breath control

——————————— WORKOUT 28 ———————————

Distance	Stroke	Time
	Choice of strokes	6:00 warm-up
200	I.M., broken	Rest :10 at each 100.
200	Free	Even pace
2 × 100	I.M.	On 2:30
		Rest :05 at each 50.
100	I.M., broken	Rest :05 after each 25.
100	Free	Negative split
2 × 50	# 1: 25 fly/25 back	On 1:15
	# 2: 25 breast/25 free	On 1:15
4 × 75	Kick: 25 fly/25 back/25 breast	On 2:00
6 × 75	Free	On 1:45
100	Free	Swim-down

1,750 yards, plus 6:00 swim, total

EMPHASIS: Individual medley conditioning; leg conditioning

─────────────── **WORKOUT 29** ───────────────

Distance	Stroke	Time
400	Free	Warm-up
	100: kick	
	100: pull	
	200: swim	
400	Pull: free	
	Breathe every 4 strokes.	
100	4th favorite stroke	Rest :20 after
75	3rd favorite stroke	each distance.
50	2nd favorite stroke	
25	Favorite stroke	
100	Free, descending	On 2:00
75		On 1:30
50		On 1:00
25		On :30
100	Fly, back, or free, descending	On 2:10
75	(all the same stroke)	On 1:40
50		On 1:10
25		On :40
4 × 100	Kick: choice of strokes	
200	Free	Swim-down

2,150 yards total
EMPHASIS: Building speed and breath control

─────────────── **WORKOUT 30** ───────────────

Distance	Stroke	Time
300	Free	Warm-up
	100: right-arm swim*	
	100: left-arm swim*	
	100: long strokes	
2 × 200	Free, progressive	On 4:00
4 × 50	Pull: free with pull buoy,	On 1:20
	paddles, and tube	
4 × 100	Back	On 2:15
	Streamline off walls.	
4 × 100	Fly, with fins	On 2:15
4 × 50	Kick: free	On 1:10
200	Free	Swim-down

2,100 yards total
EMPHASIS: General conditioning in freestyle; ankle flexibility

─────────

* See Glossary.

—————————————————— **WORKOUT 31** ——————————————————

Distance	Stroke	Time
300	I.M., reverse order of strokes 25 swim/25 kick (no board)/25 swim for each stroke	Warm-up
500	Free	Time yourself.
300	Alternate 25 back and 25 free.	
300	Alternate 25 breast and 25 free.	
5 × 50	Free, very fast	On 3:00
12 × 25	Fly	On :45
150	Free	Swim-down

2,100 yards total

EMPHASIS: Distance conditioning; speed in freestyle and butterfly

—————————————————— **WORKOUT 32** ——————————————————

Distance	Stroke	Time
450	Free, bilateral breathing	Warm-up
2 × { 150	Kick: free	Rest :30 after each 150.
150	Pull: back	
150	Swim: free	
100	Breast or fly, progressive	Rest :20 after each
75		distance.
50		
25		
9 × 50	# 1–3: 25 fly/25 back #4–6: 25 back/25 breast # 7–9: 25 breast/25 free	
150	Free	Swim-down

2,200 yards total

EMPHASIS: Arm and leg conditioning; speed in all strokes

—————— WORKOUT 33 ——————

Distance	Stroke	Time
300	Free	Warm-up
	Streamline off walls.	
3 × 100	Kick	Rest :30
	# 1: fly	
	# 2: back	
	# 3: breast	
8 × 100	Free	# 1–2 :30 rest
	Last 2 100s: very fast	# 3–4 :20 rest
		# 5–6 :10 rest
		# 7–8 :30 rest
8 × 50	Free	# 1–2 :15 rest
	Last 2 50s: very fast	# 3–4 :10 rest
		# 5–6 :05 rest
		# 7–8 :15 rest
200	Free	Swim-down

2,000 yards total
EMPHASIS: General conditioning; speed

—————— WORKOUT 34 ——————

Distance	Stroke	Time
300	Free, bilateral breathing	Warm-up
25	Pull: free	Rest :15 after each
50		distance.
75		
100		
100	Pull: choice of strokes	Rest :15 after each
75		distance.
50		
25		
50	Free	Rest :20 after each
100		distance.
150		
2 × 200		
150		
100		
50		
25	Kick: free	Rest :15 after each
50		distance.
75		
100		
100	Kick: choice	Rest :15 after each
75		distance.
50		
25		
200	Free	Swim-down

2,500 yards total
EMPHASIS: General conditioning in a variety of distances.

WORKOUT 35

Distance	Stroke	Time
200	Free, bilateral breathing	Warm-up
400	Free	Rest 1:00 after each 400.
400	Free, broken	Rest :20 after each 100.
400	Free, broken (race speed)	Rest :10 at 50s.
200	Free	Rest 1:00 at each 200.
200	Free, broken	Rest :10 at each 50.
200	Free, broken (race speed)	Rest :05 at each 25.
200	Free	Swim-down

2,200 yards total
EMPHASIS: Building race speed in middle-distance and long-distance freestyle

WORKOUT 36

Distance	Stroke	Time
200	Pull: free	Warm-up
200	Free	
400	Free Get time at 300 to beat on next swim.	Rest :30 after each distance.
300	Get time to beat at 200.	
200	Get time to beat at 100.	
100	Fast.	
2 × 200	Kick: choice of strokes	On 4:30
2 × 200	Pull: choice of strokes	On 4:00
8 × 50	# 1–2: fly # 3–4: back # 5–6: breast # 7–8: free	On 1:10
100	Free	Swim-down

2,700 yards total
EMPHASIS: Building speed over a distance; arm and leg conditioning

WORKOUT 37

Distance	Stroke	Time
400	Free, bilateral breathing	Warm-up
200	Kick: I.M.	
2 × 100	Alternate 50 fly and 50 back.	On 2:30
2 × 100	Alternate 50 back and 50 breast.	
2 × 100	Alternate 50 breast and 50 free	
2 × 100	Alternate 50 free and 50 fly.	
200	Pull: choice of strokes	

Distance	Stroke	Time
16 × 25	# 1–4: fly # 5–8: back # 9–12: breast # 13–16: free	On :40
200	Free	Swim-down

2,200 yards total

EMPHASIS: General individual medley conditioning

WORKOUT 38

Distance	Stroke	Time
500	Free 100: right-arm swim 100: left-arm swim 100: long strokes 100: ripple 100: normal	Warm-up
4 × 150	Free # 1: 50 easy/50 fast/50 fastest # 2: 50/easy/100 fast # 3: 50 fast/50 easy/50 fast # 4: 150 fast	On 2:45
4 × 125	I.M. # 1: 50 fly/25 back/ 25 breast/25 free # 2: 25 fly/50 back/ 25 breast/25 free # 3: 25 fly/ 25 back/ 50 breast/25 free # 4: 25 fly/25 back/ 25 breast/50 free	On 2:15
12 × 50	Free # 1–3: descending # 4–6: hard # 7–9: Alternate 25 easy and 25 hard. # 10–12: hard	On 1:15
200	Freestyle	Swim-down

2,400 yards total

EMPHASIS: Increasing speed

———————————————— WORKOUT 39 ————————————————

Distance	Stroke	Time
400	I.M., reverse order of strokes Alternate 50 pull and 50 kick for each stroke	Warm-up
1,650	Free Count strokes every 8 lengths, keeping number even.	Get time on each 400, keeping even pace.
200	Choice of strokes	Swim-down

2,250 yards total

EMPHASIS: Building endurance and an even pace

———————————————— WORKOUT 40 ————————————————

Distance	Stroke	Time
200	Kick: free	Warm-up
200	Pull: free	
200	Free	
10 × 100	Free # 1–5: descending # 6–10: even pace	On 2:00
5 × 50	Back	On 1:10
5 × 50	Breast	On 1:15
10 × 25	Fly Accelerate arms through the stroke.	On :50
200	Free	Swim-down

2,550 yards total

EMPHASIS: Developing a sense of pace in freestyle; building speed in butterfly

WORKOUT 41

Distance	Stroke	Time
300	Alternate 25 free and 25 choice of strokes.	Warm-up
300	I.M. Kick 2nd 25 of each stroke (without board).	Rest :45.
200	I.M. Alternate 25 kick (without board) and 25 swim of each stroke.	Rest :45.
100	I.M., fast	Rest :45.
300	Free Alternate 25 ripple and 25 normal.	Rest :30.
200	Free, with even pace. Count strokes.	Rest :30.
100	Free, very fast	Rest :30.
8 × 50	Pull: free, with pull buoy, paddles, and tube	On 1:20
8 × 50	Free, fast	On 1:05
100	Free	Swim-down

2,400 yards total

EMPHASIS: Leg conditioning in all strokes; stroke technique in freestyle

WORKOUT 42

Distance	Stroke	Time
	Choice of strokes	5:00, warm-up
400	Pull: Alternate 75 free and 25 choice of strokes.	
1,000	Free 25 easy/25 hard/50 easy/ 50 hard/75 easy/75 hard/ 100 easy/100 hard/100 easy/ 100 hard/75 easy/75 hard/ 50 easy/50 hard/25 easy/ 25 hard	
4 × 100	Back 50 kick (without board)/50 swim.	On 2:45
4 × 100	Breast 50 kick (without board)/50 swim.	On 2:50
100	Free	Swim-down

2,300 yards plus 5:00 swim total

EMPHASIS: Building endurance; arm and leg strength

WORKOUT 43

Distance	Stroke	Time
300	Free, progressive by 100s	Warm-up
6 × 150	50 fly/50 back/50 free (with fins).	On 2:45
6 × 75	Kick: choice of strokes Rest :05 after 50 and kick last 25 with face down (without breathing) as far as possible.	Rest :20 after each 75.
6 × 75	Choice of strokes (all the same stroke)	On 1:45
200	Free	Swim-down

2,300 yards total

EMPHASIS: Increasing speed; ankle flexibility; leg strength

WORKOUT 44

Distance	Stroke	Time
400	I.M., reverse order of strokes Alternate 50 kick and 50 swim for each stroke	Warm-up
400	Pull: free, with pull buoy, paddles, and tube. Breathe every 5 strokes.	
6 × 200	# 1, 3, 5: Free # 2, 4, 6: I.M. Alternate 75 your specialty and 75 your weakest stroke and 25 of each of the other two I.M. strokes.	Free on 4:00 I.M. on 4:30
4 × 50	Kick # 1: fly # 2: back # 3: breast # 4: free	On 1:10
4 × 50	# 1: fly # 2: back # 3: breast # 4: free	On 1:00
100	Free	Swim-down

2,500 yards total

EMPHASIS: Middle-distance and endurance individual medley conditioning; breath control; leg strength

WORKOUT 45

Distance	Stroke	Time
100	Back	Warm-up
	50: kick	
	50: swim	
100	Breast	
	50: kick	
	50: swim	
100	Free	
	50: kick	
	50: swim	
3 × { 100	Kick: fly	Rest :20 after each 100.
100	Pull: back	
100	Swim: free	
100	Free, easy	
8 × 100	Free; last 2 100s very fast	# 1–2 on 2:00
		# 3–4 on 1:50
		# 5–6 on 1:40
		# 7–8 on 2:00
8 × 25	# 1–2: fly	On :40
	# 3–4: back	# 3–4: back
	# 5–6: breast	# 5–6: breast
	# 7–8: free	# 7–8: free
200	Free	Swim-down

2,500 yards total

EMPHASIS: Overall sprint conditioning

WORKOUT 46

Distance	Stroke	Time
300	Alternate 25 freestyle and 25 choice of strokes.	Warm-up
300	I.M. Kick 2nd 25 of each stroke.	Rest :45
200	I.M. Kick 2nd 25 of each stroke.	Rest :45.
100	I.M., fast	Rest :45.
300	Pull: free. Breathe every 6 strokes.	Rest :45.
300	Freestyle, progressive	Rest :45.
200	Free, quality Get time at 100.	Rest :45.
100	Free Beat preceding 100 time.	Rest :45.
6 × 50	Your specialty stroke	On 1:10
200	Free	Swim-down

2,300 yards total

EMPHASIS: Variety in I.M. conditioning; speed conditioning in freestyle

--- **WORKOUT 47** ---

Distance	Stroke	Time
400	Free, bilateral breathing	Warm-up
12 × 100	Free	# 1–4: on 1:50 # 5–8: on 1:40 # 9–12: on 2:00
6 × 75	Kick: free	On 1:45. Rest :05 before last 25, then no breathing as far as possible.
16 × 25	# 1, 3, 5, 7, 9, 11, 13, 15: free, no breathing # 2, 4: fly # 6, 8: back # 10, 12: breast # 14, 16: free	On :40
200	Free	Swim-down

2,650 yards total
EMPHASIS: Endurance and pace in freestyle; leg strength; breath control

--- **WORKOUT 48** ---

Distance	Stroke	Time
450	Free 150: kick 150: pull 150: swim	Warm-up
6 × 75	Back 25: right arm 25: left arm 25: normal	On 1:45
200	Back, broken	Rest :10 after each 50.
6 × 75	Breast 25: normal 25: one pull for every kick 25: normal	On 1:45
200	Breast, broken	Rest :10 after each 50.
4 × 50	Fly	On 1:15
4 × 50	Kick: choice of strokes	On 1:15
4 × 50	Pull: choice of strokes	On 1:10
200	Free	Swim-down

2,550 yards total
EMPHASIS: Stroke technique in backstroke and breaststroke; arm and leg conditioning.

WORKOUT 49

Distance	Stroke	Time
500	Free, bilateral breathing	Warm-up
400	Free	Rest :30 after each
200	Increase speed as distance	distance.
100	decreases.	
50		
4 × 100	Kick: I.M.	On 2:15
4 × 100	Pull: free	On 1:50
8 × 50	Free, descending (# 5–8 faster than # 1–4)	On 1:00
200	Free	Swim-down

2,650 yards total

EMPHASIS: Speed in freestyle; arm and leg strength

WORKOUT 50

Distance	Stroke	Time
200	Free	Warm-up
200	I.M., reverse order	
4 × 150	I.M. # 1–3: 50 fly/25 back/ 50 breast/25 free # 4–6: 25 fly/50 back/ 25 breast/50 free	On 3:00
2 × 200	Pull: free # 1: Breathe every 5 strokes. # 2: Breathe every 7 strokes.	On 3:30
4 × 150	Free Increase speed on each 50.	On 2:45
200	Kick: I.M.	
200	Free	Swim-down

2,400 yards total

EMPHASIS: Individual medley conditioning; increasing oxygen-absorbing capability and speed

5

ADVANCED
WORKOUTS

Once you've reached a level at which you can do approximately 1 hour of strenuous interval training (at heart rates of between 60 and 80 percent of the difference between your resting and maximum heart rates) with only very short rest periods, then you'll probably feel comfortable with the workouts in this section. Also, an ability to do sets of swims using each of the four competitive strokes—butterfly, backstroke, breaststroke, and freestyle—will be helpful here.

But perhaps most important, I expect that you are interested in following an advanced program of workouts only because you want to participate in competitive events. I say this because a time commitment (not to mention an energy investment) of 1–1½ hours a day of vigorous swimming—the amount of time required by most swimmers to complete the workouts in this chapter—is sufficiently beyond the fitness level and demands some very strong motivation.

The workouts in this section have been created to help you prepare to reach a competitive level in a mixture of strokes and distances, and the yardage included in each workout is approximately 2 miles. If you want more information regarding specific kinds of competitive training I recommend my book *101 Favorite Swimming Workouts,* available through *Swim Swim* magazine, 8461 Warner Dr., Culver City, CA 90230.

If you wish to compete during only a portion of the year, your training will vary. During your off season from competition, for example, you might want to follow some intermediate level workouts or simply do some long-distance swimming, kicking, and pulling. Again, whether you are primarily at the beginning, intermediate, or advanced stage, you need not stick to one level all the time.

WORKOUT 51 *

Distance	Stroke	Time
600	Free	Warm-up
	200: kick	
	200: pull	
	200: swim	
800	Free	On 11:00
	Get time at 600 mark.	
600	Free	On 8:00
	Try to beat time of previous 600.	
	Get time at 400 mark.	
400	Free	On 5:30
	Try to beat time of previous 400.	
	Get time at 200 mark.	
200	Free, fast	
	Try to beat time of previous 200.	
25	Kick: fly	Rest :15 after each
50	Kick: back	distance.
75	Kick: breast	
100	Kick: free	
100	Kick: fly	
75	Kick: back	
50	Kick: breast	
25	Kick: free	
9 × 50	Pull: free	On :50
	# 1–3: with paddles, tube, and pull buoy	
	# 4–6: with paddles and pull buoy	
	# 7–9: with pull buoy	
200	Free	Swim-down

3,750 yards total

EMPHASIS: Preparing to hold a constant pace over a distance; leg and arm conditioning

* Note that all the workouts in this book are geared to a 25-yard pool simply because this is the most common type of facility. If you train in a meter pool, multiply time intervals by 1.1 or add 5 seconds per 50 meters, 10 seconds per 100 meters, and so on.

WORKOUT 52

Distance	Stroke	Time
500	Free, bilateral breathing	Warm-up
400	I.M., broken Descend on 1st–4th 25 of each stroke.	Rest :10 after each 25.
5 × 50	Breast	On 1:00
5 × 50	Back	On :55
5 × 50	Fly	On :50
5 × 50	Free	On :45
12 × 50	Pull: free, with paddles and tube Breathe every 6 strokes.	On :50
500 = { 200 150 100 50	Free Get time for total 500 swim.	Rest :10 after each distance.
12 × 50	Kick # 1–3: fly # 4–6: back # 7–9: breast # 10–12: free	On 1:00
100	Free	Swim-down

3,700 yards total

EMPHASIS: Endurance conditioning in all strokes; pacing in distance freestyle

WORKOUT 53

Distance	Stroke	Time
400	Free, bilateral breathing	Warm-up
16 × 100 plus 1 × 50	Free Hold a steady pace.	On 1:20
4 × 100	Kick: your specialty stroke (no fins with breast)	On 1:45
8 × 50	Free Breathe every 6 strokes.	On :50
4 × 100	Pull: your specialty stroke	On 1:30
200	Free	Swim-down

3,450 yards total

EMPHASIS: Pacing in distance freestyle; increasing lung capacity

WORKOUT 54

Distance	Stroke	Time
400	Free	Warm-up
	100: swim	
	100: pull	
	100: kick	
	100: swim	
400	I.M., reverse order of strokes	
400	I.M., progressive	
4 × 200	Choice of strokes (not free), descending. Do all the same stroke.	On 3:15
8 × 75	Pull: free	On 1:15
8 × 75	Kick: free	On 1:40
100	Free	Swim-down

3,300 yards total

EMPHASIS: General individual medley conditioning; arm and leg strength in freestyle

WORKOUT 55

Distance	Stroke	Time
500	Free, bilateral breathing	Warm-up
20 × 25	Pull: free with paddles and tube	On :30
200	Free	On 3:00
2 × 100		On 1:30
4 × 50		On :45
8 × 25		On :25
200	Your specialty stroke	On 3:15
2 × 100	(other than free)	On 1:45
4 × 50		On 1:00
8 × 25		On :45
20 × 25	Kick: free	On :30
200	Free	Swim-down

3,300 yards total

EMPHASIS: Sprint and middle distance conditioning in two strokes

───────────────── **WORKOUT 56** ─────────────────

Distance	Stroke	Time
600	Free	Warm-up
	100: right arm	
	100: left arm	
	100: catch-up*	
	100: long strokes*	
	100: ripple	
	100: normal	
3 × 300	Free, progressive	On 4:30
10 × 100	# 1: fly	On 2:00
	# 2, 4, 6, 8: I.M.	
	# 3: back	
	# 5: breast	
	# 7: free	
	# 9: 50 fly/50 back	
	# 10: 50 breast/50 free	
12 × 50	Kick: choice of strokes	On 1:00
200	Free	Swim-down

3,300 yards total

EMPHASIS: Freestyle stroke technique and conditioning; sprinting in all strokes

───────

* See Glossary.

───────────────── **WORKOUT 57** ─────────────────

Distance	Stroke	Time
400	I.M., reverse order	Warm-up
	Alternate 50 kick (no board)	
	and 50 swim.	
5 × 200	Free	# 1 on 3:20
	Hold even pace.	# 2 on 3:10
		# 3 on 3:00
		# 4 on 2:50
		# 5 on 2:40
100	Free, easy	
4 × 150	Pull: 50 fly/50 back/50 breast	On 2:30
8 × 75	25 fly/25 back/25 breast	On 1:15
4 × 100	Kick	On 2:00
	# 1: fly	
	# 2: back	
	# 3: breast	
	# 4: free	
200	Free	Swim-down

3,300 yards total

EMPHASIS: Maintaining pace in middle-distance freestyle; sprint conditioning in all strokes

WORKOUT 58

Distance	Stroke	Time
200	Free	Warm-up
150	Breast	
100	Back	
50	Fly	
200	Free, broken	500 on 7:00.
150	Get swimming time for 500.	Rest :10 after each
100		distance.
50		
200	Free, broken	500 on 7:00
100	Get time for 500 and descend.	Rest :10 after each
100		distance.
100		
200	Free, broken	500 on 7:00
100	Get time for 500 and descend.	Rest :10 after each
50		distance.
50		
50		
50		
500	Pull: free	500 on 7:00.
8 × 50	# 1–2: 25 fly/25 back	On 1:00
	# 3–4: 25 back/25 breast	
	# 5–6: 25 breast/25 free	
	# 7–8: 25 free/25 fly	
8 × 25	Your specialty stroke	On :30
	Alternate 25 hard and 25 easy.	
100	Free	Swim-down

3,200 yards total

EMPHASIS: Developing speed over a long and a short distance

WORKOUT 59

Distance	Stroke	Time
600	Free	Warm-up
	200: kick	
	200: pull	
	200: free	
6 × 200	# 1, 3, 5: free	Free on 3:00.
	# 2, 4, 6: I.M.	I.M. on 3:30.
	75 your weakest stroke/75 your	
	specialty stroke/25 of each of	
	others	
6 × 100	Pull: free, with paddles and tube	On 1:30
12 × 50	Kick: choice of strokes	On 1:00
100	Free	Swim-down

3,100 yards total

EMPHASIS: Developing your strongest and your weakest strokes; arm and leg
conditioning

WORKOUT 60

Distance	Stroke	Time
500	Free Ripple every other 25.	Warm-up
2 × 250	I.M. 100 fly/75 back/50 breast/ 25 free	Rest :30 after each 250.
2 × 250	I.M. 25 fly/50 back/75 breast/ 100 free	Rest :30 after each 250.
4 × 100	Kick: I.M., with fins Drag feet (don't kick) on breast.	On 1:50
4 × 100	I.M.	On 1:45
4 × 100	Pull: your weakest stroke	On 1:40
16 × 25	# 1–4: fly # 5–8: back # 9–12: breast # 13–16: free	On :30
200	Free	Swim-down

3,300 yards total

EMPHASIS: General sprint conditioning

WORKOUT 61

Distance	Stroke	Time
400	Free 100: swim 100: kick 100: pull 100: swim	Warm-up
8 × 50	Free Breathe every 6 strokes.	On :50
16 × 100	Free Hold even pace.	# 1–4: on 1:45 # 5–8: on 1:35 # 9–12: on 1:25 # 13–16: on 1:15
100	Choice of strokes, easy	
50 100 150 200	Pull: fly, back, or breast (all same stroke)	Rest :15 after each distance.

Distance	Stroke	Time
200	Kick: fly, back, or breast	Rest :15 after each
150	(all same stroke)	distance.
100		
50		
100	Free	Swim-down

3,600 yards total

EMPHASIS: Developing a sense of pace in distance swimming; arm and leg strength

WORKOUT 62

Distance	Stroke	Time
400	I.M., reverse order	Warm-up
	Alternate 50 kick (without board)	
	and 50 swim of each stroke	
400	Pull: I.M.	
10 × 100	I.M.	On 1:45
	Odd #: original order of I.M.	
	strokes	
	Even #: reverse order	
400	Kick: I.M., progressive by 100s	
10 × 75	25 fly/25 back/25 free, with fins	Rest :20 after each 75.
200	Free	Swim-down

3,150 yards total

EMPHASIS: General individual medley conditioning

WORKOUT 63

Distance	Stroke	Time
400	Free, bilateral breathing	Warm-up
33 × 50	Free	Rest :10 after each 50
	Get total swimming time for 1,650	
	yards (subtract the rest time of	
	5:20 from the total).	
100	Free, easy	
5 × 100	Pull: free, with paddles and tube	On 1:30
200	Free, broken; very fast	Rest :10 after each 50.
200	Your specialty stroke, broken;	Rest :10 after each 50.
	very fast	
200	Free	Swim-down

3,250 yards total

EMPHASIS: Pace and speed in freestyle

WORKOUT 64

Distance	Stroke	Time
200	Kick: choice of stroke	Warm-up
200	Pull: choice of stroke	
200	Choice of stroke	
400	Alternate 25 free and 25 fly	
4 × 50	Fly	On :55
400	Alternate 25 free and 25 back	
4 × 50	Back	On :55
400	Alternate 25 free and 25 breast	
4 × 50	Breast	On 1:00
400	Free	
4 × 50	Free	On :50
200	Free	Swim-down

3,200 yards total

EMPHASIS: Variety in endurance conditioning

WORKOUT 65

Distance	Stroke	Time
400	Free Alternate 25 ripple and 25 long strokes.	Warm-up
400	I.M. 100 of each stroke. Descend 2nd 50 of each stroke.	
5 × 200	Back	On 3:00
400	Pull: free. Breathe every 6 strokes.	
5 × 100	Fly, with fins	On 1:30
400	Kick: I.M.	
5 × 50	Breast	On 1:00
200	Free	Swim-down

3,550 yards total

EMPHASIS: General middle-distance and sprint conditioning

WORKOUT 66

Distance	Stroke	Time
200	Free	Warm-up
150	Breast	
100	Back	
50	Fly	
5 × 100	Pull	Rest :20 after each 100.
	# 1: fly	
	# 2: back	
	# 3: breast	
	# 4: free	
	# 5: I.M.	
10 × 50	Free, very fast	On 1:00
5 × 100	# 1: fly	On 1:45
	# 2: back	
	# 3: breast	
	# 4: free	
	# 5: I.M.	
10 × 50	Your specialty stroke (not free)	On 1:00
5 × 100	Kick	Rest :20 after each 100.
	# 1: fly	
	# 2: back	
	# 3: breast	
	# 4: free	
	# 5: I.M.	
100	Free	Swim-down

3,100 yards total

EMPHASIS: Increasing arm and leg strength, building speed

WORKOUT 67

Distance	Stroke	Time
100	Free	Warm-up
100	Free, ripple	
100	Free, long strokes	
100	Free, catch-up	
100	Free	
8 × 200	Free, descend	# 1–2 on 3:00
		# 3–4 on 2:50
		# 5–6 on 2:40
		# 7–8 on 3:00
4 × 100	Pull: free, with paddles and tube	On 1:45
	# 1: Breathe every 3 strokes.	
	# 2: Breathe every 4 strokes.	
	# 3: Breathe every 5 strokes.	
	# 4: Breathe every 6 strokes.	
4 × 100	Fly, back, or breast	On 1:40
	(Choose one stroke.)	
8 × 50	25 choice of strokes/25 free	On :50
100	Free	Swim-down

3,400 yards total

EMPHASIS: Improving stroke mechanics and maintaining pace in freestyle; breath control

---
WORKOUT 68

Distance	Stroke	Time
400	Free, bilateral breathing	Warm-up
275	Free, broken	Rest :30 after 275, 250,
250	Get time for 1,650 by subtracting	225, 200, and 175;
225	3:45 (rest time) from total time	rest :15 after 150,
200		125, 100, 75, and
175		50.
1,650 { 150		
125		
100		
75		
50		
25		
10 × 75	25 fly/25 back/25 breast	On 1:20
200	Free	Swim-down

3,000 yards total

EMPHASIS: Endurance conditioning; speed in butterfly, backstroke, and breaststroke

─────────────── **WORKOUT 69** ───────────────

Distance	Stroke	Time
	Choice of strokes	6:00 warm-up
4 × 125	Kick: free	On 2:15
		Rest :10 at 100 and kick with head down (no breathing) as far as possible.
6 × 150	Alternate 50 fly/50 back/50 breast	On 2:30
12 × 50	Free, descend	# 1–3 on :50
		# 4–6 on :45
		# 7–9 on :40
		# 10–12 on 1:00
500	Pull: free, with paddles and tube	
8 × 25	Free	On :30
	No breathing on even 25s.	
100	Free	Swim-down

2,800 yards plus 6:00 total
EMPHASIS: Arm, leg, and sprint conditioning

─────────────── **WORKOUT 70** ───────────────

Distance	Stroke	Time
200	Free	Warm-up
150	Your weakest stroke	
100	Your specialty stroke	
50	Free	
300	Fly	Rest :30.
3 × 100	Pull: fly	On 1:45
4 × 75	Kick: fly	On 1:30
300	Back	Rest :30.
3 × 100	Pull: back	On 1:45
4 × 75	Kick: back	On 1:30
300	Breast	Rest :30
3 × 100	Pull: breast	On 2:00
4 × 75	Kick: breast	On 1:30
6 × 50	Free, very fast	On 1:30
200	Free	Swim-down

3,700 yards total
EMPHASIS: General conditioning in a variety of strokes and distances

————————— WORKOUT 71 —————————

Distance	Stroke	Time
400	Free, bilateral breathing. Count strokes every 4th 25, and keep count consistent for even pace.	Warm-up
2 × 400	Pull # 1: I.M. # 2: Free	On 6:00
4 × 200	Back	On 3:15.
3 × 200	Breast	On 3:30
2 × 200	Free	On 3:00
200	Fly	
200	Free	Swim-down

3,400 yards total

EMPHASIS: General middle-distance conditioning in all strokes

————————— WORKOUT 72 —————————

Distance	Stroke	Time
600	Free 200: kick 200: pull 200: swim	Warm-up
400	I.M. Descend 1st–4th 25 of each stroke	Rest :05 after each 25.
100	Free Do as many 100s as you can until you can't make the interval. Then do 2 more 100s on last interval made.	Best time for 100 + :40 = 1st interval. Subtract :05 more on each subsequent interval.
400	Kick: I.M.	
1,000	Free for time	
100	Free	Swim-down

2,500 yards, plus 100s, total

EMPHASIS: Building endurance in individual medley and freestyle

━━━━━━━━━━ WORKOUT 73 ━━━━━━━━━━

Distance	Stroke	Time
400	Free, bilateral breathing	Warm-up
50	Free	On :50
	Build speed from 50 to 200.	
100		On 1:40
150		On 2:30
200		On 3:00
200		On 3:00
150		On 2:30
100		On 1:40
50		On :50
8 x 75	Pull: free, with paddles and tube	On 1:20
8 x 100	I.M.	On 1:45
8 x 75	# 1–4: your specialty stroke	On 1:30
	# 5–8: your weakest stroke	
200	Free	Swim-down

3,600 yards total

EMPHASIS: Building speed, individual medley conditioning; leg strength in two strokes, arm strength against resistance

━━━━━━━━━━ WORKOUT 74 ━━━━━━━━━━

Distance	Stroke	Time
600	Free	Warm-up
	300: pull	
	200: kick	
	100: swim	
5 x 200	Free, even pace	On 3:00
400	Kick: I.M.	
400	Pull: I.M.	
400	I.M.	
10 x 100	Choice of strokes (not free)	On 1:30
100	Free	Swim-down

3,900 yards total

EMPHASIS: Distance conditioning for even pace

—————————————— **WORKOUT 75** ——————————————

Distance	Stroke	Time
500	Free, bilateral breathing	Warm-up
3 × 300	100 fly/100 back/100 breast	On 4:30
4 × 200	I.M.	On 3:30
5 × 100	I.M.	On 1:40
6 × 50	Free	On :50
100	Pull: free, with paddles and tube	Rest :20.
75		Rest :15.
50		Rest :10.
25		Rest :05.
100	Kick: choice of strokes	Rest :20.
75		Rest :15.
50		Rest :10.
25		Rest :05.
200	Free	Swim-down

3,700 yards total

EMPHASIS: Individual medley conditioning; arm and leg conditioning

6

WORKOUTS THAT EMPHASIZE VARIETY

During the course of your swim training, there may be times when you feel you need a change of pace. But rather than take time completely away from swimming, you may find that changing the format of your workouts for a day, a week, or longer will provide you with the needed refreshment.

The workouts contained in this section provide you with an opportunity for conditioning and skill development while also contributing relief from some weeks or months of more intensive interval training so that you may return to your regular training relaxed and stimulated without the sensation—physical or mental—that you've somehow lost time.

The following are some methods, some borrowed and some self-conceived, that I have used to lend interest and variety during training:

Around-the-Walls 50s: You will get more practice on your turns if you begin and end your 50s in the middle of the pool rather than at the wall because you will be doing two turns per 50 yards (in a 25-yard pool) rather than just one.

Backstroke Kick with Perpendicular Arm or Arms: As you kick on your back, hold one arm perpendicular to the surface of the

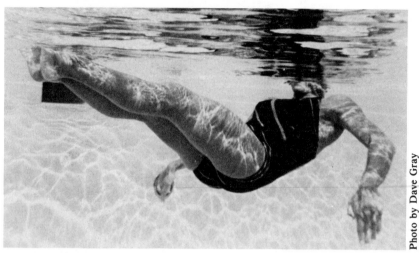

Photo by Dave Gray

Feet-first breaststroke

water in a position resembling the midpoint of a regular arm recovery. Your other arm should be resting on the water and extended directly behind your head. Once you can satisfactorily kick a length of the pool in this position, try holding both arms straight up in the air.

Feet-First Breaststroke Pull: Your body should be in a right-angle position with your hips down in the water and your ankles and ears above the surface. Propulsion comes from taking small

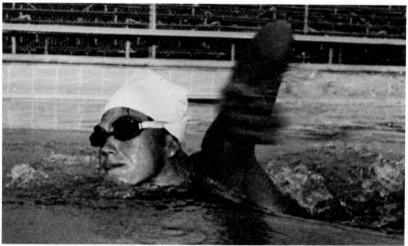

Photo by Dave Gray

Head-out freestyle

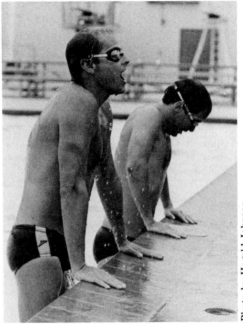

Press-ups

Photo by Harald Johnson

breaststroke pulls at your sides so that your body moves forward feet first.

Head-Out Freestyle: Swim freestyle for short sprints with your head out, focusing your eyes on a point directly in front of you, and don't let your head move from side to side with the motion of your strokes. You should not attempt this exercise until you have good solid stroke mechanics in freestyle, since holding your head too high can become a habit.

Mixed strokes: Do the arm pull of one stroke and the kick of another at the same time. (For example, do the freestyle arm pull while doing the breaststroke kick.)

Press-Ups: Begin by placing your hands, shoulder width apart, flat on the edge of the pool while allowing your body to rest in a vertical position in deep water. (If water deeper than your height isn't available, try bending your knees in this position in shallower water.) Then press your body up out of the water until your elbows are locked. Return to the starting position. You may wish to drape a towel over the edge of the pool to avoid abrasion to your wrists and rubbing the front of your suit.

Porpoise: From a prone position on the surface of the water,

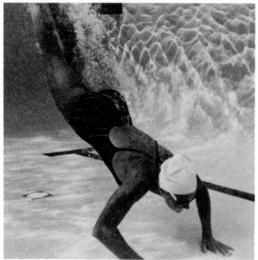

Porpoise (going down)

Photo by Dave Gray

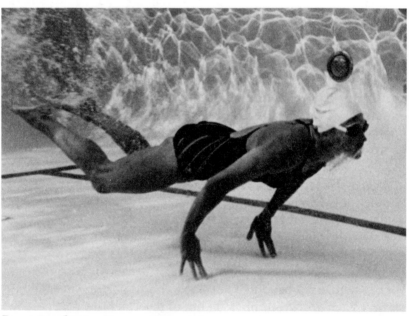

Porpoise (beginning to come up)

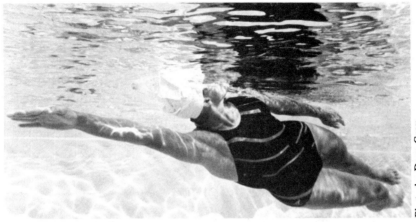

Side freestyle kick

butterfly kick your way to the bottom of the pool (if the water is about 6 feet deep or less), touching it with your hands. Then place your feet where your hands touched, raising your arms above your head in streamline position and push off at a 45° angle toward the surface. Once you reach the surface, grab a quick breath of air and repeat the maneuver.

Side Butterfly or Freestyle Kick: Do your butterfly or freestyle kicking on your side rather than your stomach and extend one arm directly under your ear. You may hold a kickboard under your forearm for support if you wish. The other arm is stretched out along your side on top of your body.

Swimming in Place: You will need an 18–20-foot length of surgical tubing with a diameter of ½ inch, and a sturdy, preferably wide, canvas belt. Make a loop at each end of the tubing to a stationary object near the edge of the pool and slip the belt around the waist. Then swim out from the edge as far as the tubing will allow, and keep stroking to avoid slipping backward.

Swimming in place

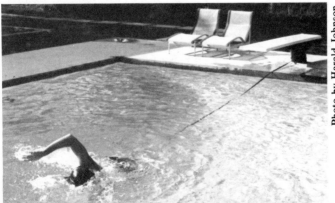

Vertical Kicking: Kick with a breaststroke or eggbeater kick (a breaststroke kick but with one leg at a time) in a completely vertical position with your hands elevated above the surface or on top of your head. The higher out of the water you can bring your body with the force of your kick, the greater the training benefit.

The following workouts have been constructed with the intention of providing variety in training along with the opportunity for development of skills using the methods described in this chapter.

───────────────WORKOUT 76*───────────────

Distance	Stroke	Time
100	Free, bilateral breathing	Warm-up
100	Side free kick**	
100	Choice of strokes	
100	Side fly kick**	
4 × 100	Back 25 right arm only/25 left arm only/25 with legs crossed (no kick)/25 normal	Rest :20 after each 100.
400	Pull: free Breathe every 3 strokes on 1st 100, every 4 on 2nd, every 5 on 3rd, every 6 on 4th.	

	Kick
	   # 1: fly
	   # 2: back
	   # 3: breast
	   # 4: free
		4 × 2:15
		   :45 hard/:15 moderate/:30 hard/:15 moderate/:15 hard/:15 moderate
		Rest :30 after each 2:15.

8 × 50	Mixed strokes
	   # 1–2: breast pull with free kick
	   # 3–4: back pull with fly kick
	   # 5–6: free pull with breast kick
	   # 7–8: fly pull (on back) with back kick
		Rest :20 after each 50.

400	I.M., with fins (let feet drag on breast)	
200	Free	Swim-down

2,200 yards, plus 9:00 kick, total

EMPHASIS: Developing propulsion on up-and-down phase of freestyle kick and butterfly kick; learning to push through the end of the stroke in backstroke; building lung capacity, coordination, and leg strength

---

* Note that all the workouts in this book are geared to a 25-yard pool simply because this is the most common type of facility. If you train in a meter pool, multiply time intervals by 1.1 or add 5 seconds per 50 meters, 10 seconds per 100 meters, and so on.
** See page 63.

WORKOUT 77

Distance	Stroke	Time
500	Free	Warm-up
500	Alternate 50 free and 25 porpoise* and 25 fly. Up to 50 press-ups*	No longer than 5:00
500	Mixed strokes (must do each 50 a different stroke than the preceding 50). Up to 50 press-ups	No longer than 5:00
500	Free Wear T-shirt or shorts over your swim suit.	
200	Free	Swim-down

2,200 yards, plus press-ups, total

EMPHASIS: Practicing the undulating motion necessary for an efficient butterfly; strengthening the arms for the final phase of freestyle, backstroke, and butterfly pulls; general strengthening and conditioning through the use of drag

_____

* See page 61.

WORKOUT 78

Distance	Stroke	Time
	Choice of strokes	10:00 warm-up
8 × 50	Kick: choice of strokes Stop in middle of pool on 1st 25 and hold board above surface, kicking vertically* for :05.	Rest :15 after each 50.
2 × 25	Feet-first breaststroke pull**	Rest :30 after each 25.
4 × 250	25 choice of strokes/100 free/ 25 choice of strokes/ 100 free	Rest :45 after each 250.
8 × 50	Around-the-walls 50s*** Choice of strokes	Rest :15 after each 50.
2 × 25	Feet-first breaststroke pull**	Rest :30 after each 25.
4 × 125	Head-out freestyle on 1st, 3rd, and 5th 25s.	Rest :30 after each 125.
200	Free	Swim-down

2,600 yards, plus 10:00 warm-up, total

EMPHASIS: Building leg strength and coordination into the kick; strengthening the abdominal muscles and triceps for the purpose of increasing efficiency in pushing against water; improving turns

_____

* See page 64.
** See page 60.
*** See page 59.

WORKOUT 79

Distance	Stroke	Time
250	Kick: choice of strokes	Warm-up
250	Pull: choice of strokes	
250	Choice of strokes	
6 x 75	Fly	Rest :20 after each 75.
	25 kick/25 pull/25 swim	
6 x 75	Back	Rest :20 after each 75.
	25 kick/25 pull/25 swim	
6 x 75	Breast	Rest :20 after each 75.
	25 kick/25/pull/25 swim	
	Up to 25 press-ups	No longer than 2:00
4 x 125	Kick: choice of strokes with fins (no board)	Rest :30 after each 125.
250	Free	Swim-down

2,850 yards, plus press-ups, total

EMPHASIS: General leg and arm conditioning in butterfly, backstroke, and breaststroke; ankle flexibility; building tricep strength

WORKOUT 80

Distance	Stroke	Time
1,000	Alternate 75 free and 25 stroke of choice	Warm-up
	Free	4 x 3:00
	Swimming in place*	Rest 1:00 after each 3:00.
4 x 125	Kick	Rest :30 after each 125.
	Alternate 25 breast with hands at sides and 25 back with arms extended behind head	
1,000	Pull: choice of strokes	
	Up to 50 press-ups	No longer than 5:00

2,500 yards, plus 12:00 and press-ups, total

EMPHASIS: Swimming against high resistance to build general strength; conditioning and balance in breaststroke; backstroke kicking; endurance conditioning; and building arm strength

---

* See page 63.

WORKOUT 81

Distance	Stroke	Time
500	Breast 100: swim 100: kick 100: pull 100: 2 kicks per pull 100: swim	Warm-up
500	Alternate 25 breast and 25 free.	
4 × 25	Porpoise	Rest :20 after each 25.
	Swimming in place Alternate 25 breast and 25 free.	2 × 3:00. Rest 1:00 after each 3:00.
4 × 25	Pull: back, with legs crossed (no pull buoy)	Rest :20 after each 25.
500	Alternate 25 fly and 25 back, with fins	
4 × 25	Back kick with perpendicular arm(s)*	Rest :20 after each 25.
10 × 50	Kick Alternate 25 fly underwater and 25 back, with fins.	Rest :20 after each 50.
200	Free	Swim-down

2,500 yards, plus 6:00 of swimming in place, total

EMPHASIS: Developing arm and leg strength and stretch forward with arms in breaststroke; undulating motion in butterfly; body position, leg strength, and timing in backstroke

---

* See page 59.

──────── WORKOUT 82 ────────

Distance	Stroke	Time
5 × 100	Free Alternate 25 head-out and 25 head down.	Warm-up Rest :10 after each 100.
500	I.M. 75 of each stroke 50 of each stroke	 Rest :20 after each 75. Rest :10 after each 50.
	Kick: choice of stroke, for distance	6:00
500	Pull: free, with paddles, tube, and shorts.	
	Choice of stroke Swim for distance	12:00
6 widths	Kicking underwater (no breathing if possible)	
200	Free	Swim-down

1,700 yards, plus 6:00 kick and 12:00 swim and 6 widths, total
EMPHASIS: Swimming with added resistance; overloading the arms and the legs
to build strength; limiting breathing during kicking to increase lung
capacity

──────── WORKOUT 83 ────────

Distance	Stroke	Time
400	Free Alternate 50 kick and 50 swim	Warm-up
4 × 25	Feet-first breast pull	Rest :30 after each 25.
	Up to 50 press-ups	No longer than 5:00
4 × 150	100 I.M. plus 25 your strongest stroke/25 your weakest stroke	Rest :40 after each 150.
4 × 150	With fins 50 porpoise/50 fly/50 porpoise	Rest :40 after each 150.
	Up to 50 press-ups	No longer than 5:00
400	Free, with T-shirt	
4 × 100	# 1: 50 fly/50 back # 2: 50 back/50 breast # 3: 50 breast/50 free # 4: 50 free/50 fly	Rest :30 after each 100.
100	Free	Swim-down

2,600 yards total plus press-ups
EMPHASIS: Increasing tricep and abdominal muscle strength; general sprint conditioning; improving undulating motion in butterfly

─────────────── **WORKOUT 84** ───────────────

Distance	Stroke	Time
200	Free	Warm-up
200	Kick: choice of stroke, with fins	
200	Choice of stroke	
	Fly, swimming in place	2 x 2:00
		Rest :45 after each
		2:00.
4 x 50	Side fly kick, with fins	Rest :15 after each 50.
2 x 2:00	Back, swimming in place	Rest :45 after each
		2:00.
4 x 50	Back kick, with fins	Rest :15 after each 50.
6 x 100	50 breast/50 free	Rest :30 after each 100.
300	Pull: free	
	100: Breathe every 3 strokes.	
	100: Breathe every 5 strokes.	
	100: Breathe every 7 strokes.	
100	Free	Swim-down

2,000 yards plus 8:00 swimming in place

EMPHASIS: Building strength against resistance, ankle flexibility, increasing your oxygen absorbing capacity

─────────────── **WORKOUT 85** ───────────────

Distance	Stroke	Time
	Choice of strokes (combination swim and kick)	10:00 warm-up
1,000	Free	
	25 easy/25 hard/50 easy/	
	50 hard/75 easy/75 hard/	
	100 easy/100 hard/100 easy/	
	100 hard/75 easy/75 hard/	
	50 easy/50 hard/25 easy/	
	25 hard	
10 x 50	Around-the-walls 50s	Rest :15 after each 50.
	# 1, 3, 5, 7, 9: back	
	# 2, 4, 6, 8, 10: breast	
4 x :30	Vertical kicking	Rest :15 after each :30
		of kicking.
20 x 25	Alternate 25 porpoise and 25 fly	Rest :15 after each 25.
100	Free	Swim-down

2,100 yards, plus 10:00 warm-up and 2:00 kick, total

EMPHASIS: Building a feel for the water as well as a sense of pace; practicing backstroke and breaststroke turns; building leg strength; working on the undulating movement in butterfly

—————————————— WORKOUT 86 ——————————————

Distance	Stroke	Time
600	Free 200: kick, with fins 200: pull, with fins 200: free, with fins	Warm-up
2 × 200	Kick, with fins # 1: side free kick # 2: side fly kick	Rest :30 after each 200.
2 × 200	Free 50: Breathe every 2 strokes. 50: Breathe every 4 strokes. 50: Breathe every 6 strokes. 50: Breathe every 8 strokes.	Rest :30 after each 200.
2 × 200	Pull: choice of mixed strokes, with paddles, tube, and shorts.	Rest :30 after each 200.
2 × 200	Mixed strokes # 1: back arms with fly kick # 2: free arms with breast kick	Rest :30 after each 200.
8 × 25	Kick with fins: fly Alternate 3 kicks underwater (without board) and 3 normal kicks on surface.	Rest :10 after each 25.
200	Free	Swim-down

2,600 yards total

EMPHASIS: Building ankle flexibility; improving coordination; developing an undulating motion in butterfly

WORKOUT 87

Distance	Stroke	Time
400	Free Alternate 50 swim and 50 kick.	Warm-up
4 x 150	Free 50 long strokes/50 ripple/ 50 normal	Rest :20 after each 150.
	Vertical kicking	4 x :30. Rest :30 after every 30 seconds of kicking.
400	Pull Alternate 25 free and 25 choice of strokes.	
4 x 100	Fly Alternate 25 fly and 25 porpoise	Rest :20 after each 100.
8 x 50	Around-the-walls 50s # 1–2: fly # 3–4: back # 5–6: breast # 7–8: free	Rest :10 after each 50.
200	Free	Swim-down

2,400 yards, plus 1:20 kick, total
EMPHASIS: Developing freestyle stroke technique; conditioning arms and legs; increasing efficiency of your turns

WORKOUT 88

Distance	Stroke	Time
500	Back 100: swim 100: kick 100: right arm 100: left arm 100: swim	Warm-up
250	Back Alternate 25 right arm and 25 left arm.	
250	Pull: back, with paddles	
500	Alternate 25 free and 25 back.	
500	Pull: free, with paddles, tube, shorts, and T-shirt	
2 x 250	50 free/200 I.M.	Rest :40 after each 250.
200	Free	Swim-down

2,700 yards total
EMPHASIS: Improving backstroke technique; building endurance

WORKOUT 89

Distance	Stroke	Time
100	Free	Warm-up
100	Pull: free	
100	Kick: side free	
100	Choice of strokes	
100	Pull: choice of strokes	
100	Kick: side fly	
4 × 25	Porpoise	Rest :15 after each 25.
4 × 100	Fly, with fins	Rest :30 after each 100.
4 × 25	Fly kick on your back, with fins	Rest :15 after each 25.
4 × 100	Back, with fins	Rest :30 after each 100.
4 × 25	Feet-first breast	Rest :15 after each 25.
4 × 100	Breast 2 kicks for every pull on every other 25	Rest :30 after each 100.
4 × 25	Head-out free	Rest :15 after each 25.
4 × 100	Free: Count the number of strokes each length and keep the stroke count consistent.	Rest :30 after each 100.
200	Free	Swim-down

2,800 yards total

EMPHASIS: General short-distance conditioning and sharpening up of all strokes

WORKOUT 90

Distance	Stroke	Time
500	Any combination of strokes, kicking, and pulling	Warm-up
1,000	Free: Alternate 50 moderate and 50 fast.	

500	Pull: free
	For each 100—
	    25: Breathe every 3 strokes.
	    25: Breathe every 5 strokes.
	    25: Breathe every 7 strokes.
	    25: Breathe every 9 strokes.	

5 × 100	Kick # 1: 50 fly/50 back # 2: 50 back/50 breast # 3: 50 breast/50 free # 4: 50 free/50 fly	Rest :30 after each 100.
4 × 25	Head-out free	Rest :15 after each 25.
200	Free	Swim-down

2,800 yards total

EMPHASIS: Endurance conditioning in freestyle; building leg strength in all strokes

7

CREATING YOUR OWN WORKOUTS

Once you've gained some understanding of workout organization and you've had a chance to discover which aspects of your training you wish to spend additional time on, it's fun to try your hand at inventing your own workouts. The following skeleton workouts have been constructed to give you some guidance and also to afford you the opportunity to use your own knowledge and creativity.

The workout suggestions are made here according to total distance of a particular type of training, the number of minutes to be spent in each area, the percentage of the total training time you allot for different types of conditioning, or the number of repeat swims you do. Where stroke, distance, or interval are not indicated, choose your own and fill in the blank. In this way you will have the opportunity to determine the emphasis of each workout. When you finish adding whatever you need to the workouts in this chapter, each set of swims should designate the stroke, the distance, the number of repeat swims, the time interval, and the emphasis as well as any special equipment needed to complete the exercise.

Have fun, coach!

─────────WORKOUT 91 *─────────

Distance	Stroke	Time
400		Warm-up
800	Choose stroke, distance, and intervals. Distance should be a minimum of 100 yards per swim.	

400	Pull
	    Choose number of strokes
	        per breath.	

800	Choose stroke and intervals. Distance per swim should be less than above.	
400	Kick	
200		Swim-down
3,000	yards total	

EMPHASIS:

_____

* Note that all the workouts in this book are geared to a 25-yard pool simply because this is the most common type of facility. If you train in a meter pool, multiply time intervals by 1.1 or add 5 seconds per 50 meters, 10 seconds per 100 meters, and so on.

─────────── WORKOUT 92 ───────────

Distance	Stroke	Time
		6:00 warm-up
	Build speed from the beginning of each swim to the end.	8:00
	Use at least 2 different strokes. Long rest; high speed.	16:00
	Kick	8:00
	Practice on turns; use all strokes	6:00
	Short distances (50s or 25s)	8:00
		3:00 swim-down
_____	yards total (55:00)	

EMPHASIS:

WORKOUT 93

Distance	Stroke	Time
300		Warm-up
300	Choose short distances; limit breathing.	
300	Kicks	
1,000	Free, for distance. Choose distance and intervals.	
300	Pull, with paddles	
300	Choose stroke: sprint	
200		Swim-down
2,700	yards total	

EMPHASIS:

WORKOUT 94

Distance (Percentage)	Stroke	Time
15%		Warm-up
20%	Alternate fast and moderate swimming.	
40%	Distance swimming	
10%	Kick	
10%	Pull	
5%		Swim-down
_____	yards total	

EMPHASIS:

WORKOUT 95

Distance	Stroke	Time
400		Warm-up
400	I.M.s	
800	Frees	
400	Pulls	
400	Kicks	
200		Swim-down
2,600	yards total	

EMPHASIS:

───── WORKOUT 96 ─────

Distance	Stroke	Time
		5:00 warm-up
	Do all strokes	12:00
	Kick	5:00
	Middle distance repeats	20:00
	Pull	5:00
		5:00 swim-down

_____ yards total (52:00)

EMPHASIS:

───── WORKOUT 97 ─────

Distance	Stroke	Time
450		Warm-up
3 × 300		On
3 × 150		On
12 × 75		On
12 × 25		On
150		Swim-down

3,150 yards total

EMPHASIS:

───── WORKOUT 98 ─────

Distance (Percentage)	Stroke	Time
15%		Warm-up
30%	Distance training: Choose stroke	
25%	Middle distance training: Choose a different stroke than above.	
15%	Kick, sprint	
10%	Sprint	
5%		Swim-down

_____ yards total

EMPHASIS:

WORKOUT 99

Distance	Stroke	Time
400		Warm-up
800		
400		
800		
400		
200		Swim-down

3,000 yards total

EMPHASIS:

WORKOUT 100

Distance	Stroke	Time
		5:00 warm-up
	Free stroke drills	10:00
	Kick: choose stroke	7:00
	Pull: free	7:00
	Interval swimming using your specialty stroke	20:00
		3:00 swim-down

_____ yards (52:00) total

EMPHASIS:

WORKOUT 101

Distance	Stroke	Time
400		Warm-up
4 × 200		On
400		
8 × 100		On
4 × 50		On
200		Swim-down

2,800 yards total

EMPHASIS:

―――――――――――――**WORKOUT 102**―――――――――――

Distance (Percentage)	Stroke	Time
10%		Warm-up
20%	Stroke drills: your weakest stroke	
15%	Pull: choose stroke	
30%	I.M.s	
15%	Kick: choose stroke	
10%		Swim-down

_____ yards total

EMPHASIS:

―――――――――――――**WORKOUT 103**―――――――――――

Distance	Stroke	Time
	Alternate 25 ripple and 25 long strokes	Warm-up
	Stroke drills: your specialty stroke	
	Fly or back	
	Pull, with paddles	
	Back or breast	
	Kick: free sprint	
	Free sprint, limiting breathing	
		Swim-down

_____ yards total

EMPHASIS:

WORKOUT 104

Distance	Stroke	Time
300		Warm-up
400		
2 × 400		On
600		
8 × 25		On
4 × 100		On
8 × 25		On
100		Swim-down

3,000 yards total

EMPHASIS:

WORKOUT 105

Distance	Stroke	Time
	Pull, with paddles and tube	
	Alternate 25 choice of strokes and 25 free.	
	Distance free	
	Kick	
	Alternate 25 your specialty stroke and 25 your weakest stroke.	
	Free, sprint	Swim-down

_____ yards total

EMPHASIS:

8

TRAINING IN A POOL FOR OPEN WATER SWIMMING

Because distances in the open water are not accurately measurable and conditions can vary greatly, the best place to develop cardiovascular conditioning is in the pool. As is discussed in Chapter 9, for reasons of familiarizing yourself with the environment in which you will be racing, you'll want to do some training directly in the open water. But for conditioning, nothing beats pool training.

Some adaptations, however, can be made to your pool workouts to make them more specific in building skills useful in open water swimming.

First, since racing in the open water generally requires some hard sprinting at the very beginning to get away from the crowd, I have introduced within the workouts in this chapter some sets in which the first swim in a series is the fastest rather than the slowest, as it is in a descending progression of swims.

Second, I have for the most part set up the workouts in ¼-mile, ½-mile, and full-mile increments rather than around distances found in pool competition. The reason for this is that most open water swims are measured in miles, not in yards.

Third, the total distances of the workouts contained in this section are greater than those in other sections because the shortest

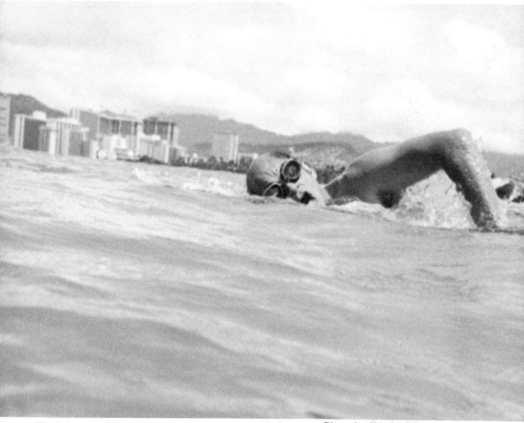

Training in open water   Photo by Harald Johnson

open water swims are usually at least one mile, whereas the longest
pool event is just under a mile, so the extra distance per workout
is helpful for conditioning. As you're doing distance training,
count the number of strokes you take per length, making an effort
to gain the greatest distance per stroke. If your number of strokes
is consistent, you can be quite sure that your pace will be even as
well.

Finally, the workouts in this chapter are all freestyle workouts.
And I expect you will want to emphasize freestyle in your training
for open water since, for most people, it's the fastest stroke, and
the best way to gain efficiency and speed in a stroke is to *do* that
stroke. At the same time, for variety, you'll probably sometimes
want to do those workouts in the other chapters that include other
strokes.

─────────────WORKOUT 106*─────────────

Distance	Stroke	Time
150	Kick: free	Warm-up
150	Pull: free	
150	Free	
18 x 100	Free	Rest :10 after each 100.
9 x 50	Pull: free	On 1:00
5 x 50	Head-out: free	On 1:10
6 x 75	Kick: free	On 2:00
	Rest :05 before last 25, then kick with head down (no breathing) as far as possible.	
150	Free	Swim-down

3,550 yards total

EMPHASIS: Endurance and even pacing; arm and leg strength, improving oxygen absorbing capabilities

───────

* Note that all the workouts in this book are geared to a 25-yard pool simply because this is the most common type of facility. If you train in a meter pool, multiply time intervals by 1.1 or add 5 seconds per 50 meters, 10 seconds per 100 meters, and so on.

─────────────WORKOUT 107─────────────

Distance	Stroke	Time
200	Free	Warm-up
250	Free	
	Alternate 50 hard and 50 easy.	
9 x 100	Pull: free, with paddles and tube	On 2:00
9 x 50	Free	Rest :10 after each 50.
	Breathe on your least favorite side.	
9 x 50	Free, bilateral breathing	Rest :15 after each 50.
9 x 50	Free	Rest :20 after each 50.
	Breathe every 6 strokes.	
9 x 100	Kick, free	On 2:15
100	Free	Swim-down

3,700 yards total

EMPHASIS: Short distance pacing; developing breathing technique on both sides; breath control

WORKOUT 108

Distance	Stroke	Time
450	Free	Warm-up
	Alternate 50 swim and 50 kick.	
3 × 450	Free	Rest :30 after each 450.
450	Kick: free, with fins	
450	Pull: free, with paddles and tube	
3 × 450	Free	Rest :30 after each 450.
150	Free	Swim-down

4,200 yards total

EMPHASIS: Endurance; ankle flexibility; upper body conditioning

WORKOUT 109

Distance	Stroke	Time
100	Free, right arm	Warm-up
100	Free, left arm	
100	Free, ripple	
100	Free, long strokes	
9 × 200	Free	On 4:00
	Sprint 1st and 6th 200; even pace on all others	
4 × 100	Pull: free, with paddles and tube	On 2:00
4 × 100	Kick: free with face in water	On 2:10
	Breathe every 6 downbeats.	
200	Free	Swim-down

3,200 yards total

EMPHASIS: Stroke technique; sprinting; increasing lung capacity

WORKOUT 110

Distance	Stroke	Time
	Choice of strokes	6:00 warm-up
5 × 100	Kick: free, with fins	On 1:45
100	Free	Rest :10.
200	100: fast	Rest :20.
300	200 and 400: bilateral breathing	Rest :30.
400		Rest :40.
500		Rest :50.
5 × 100	Pull: free	On 2:00
	Breathe every 8 strokes.	
250	Free	Swim-down

2,750 yards, plus 6:00 swim, total

EMPHASIS: Developing leg strength, ability to breathe on both sides, and lung capacity

─────────────────────**WORKOUT 111**─────────

Distance	Stroke	Time
225	Kick: free	Warm-up
225	Free	
900	Free, bilateral breathing	
10 × 25	Head-out: free	On :40
900	Pull: free, with paddles	
10 × 25	Kick: free	On :40
250	Free	Swim-down

3,000 yards total

EMPHASIS: Practicing technique used to sight markers in open water; arm and leg conditioning

─────────────────────**WORKOUT 112**─────────

Distance	Stroke	Time
50	Free	Warm-up
100	Kick: free	
150	Pull: free	
200	Free	
25	Pull: free, with paddles and tube	Rest :05.
50		Rest :10.
75		Rest :15.
100		Rest :20.
100		Rest :20.
75		Rest :15.
50		Rest :10.
25		Rest :05.
1,800	Free 25 easy/25 hard/ 50 easy/ 50 hard/75 easy/75 hard/ 100 easy/100 hard/125 easy/ 125 hard/150 easy/150 hard/ 175 easy/175 hard/200 easy/ 200 hard	
25	Kick: free	Rest :05.
50		Rest :10.
75		Rest :15.
100		Rest :20.
100		Rest :20.
75		Rest :15.
50		Rest :10.
25		Rest :05.
200	Free	Swim-down

3,500 yards total

EMPHASIS: General endurance conditioning at different speeds; variety

―――――――――――――――WORKOUT 113――――――――――――――――

Distance	Stroke	Time
200	Free	Warm-up
200	Free	
	Alternate 25 head-out and	
	25 normal	
4 × 100	Free	100s on 1:40
2 × 200		200s on 3:15
400		Rest :30 between
		distances.
8 × 50	Kick: free	On 1:05
4 × 100	Pull: free, with paddles	100s on 1:50
2 × 200		200s on 3:45
400		Rest :30 between
		distances.
200	Free	Swim-down

3,400 yards total

EMPHASIS: Developing speed early in a swim; practicing lifting head; arm and leg conditioning

―――――――――――――――WORKOUT 114――――――――――――――――

Distance	Stroke	Time
450	Free, stroke bilateral breathing	Warm-up
9 × 50	Free	On 1:00
	No breathing 5 yards before and	
	after each wall	
9 × 100	Free	On 2:00
	# 1, 4, 7: Fast	
	# 2, 5, 8: Breathe on your least	
	favorite side	
	# 3, 6, 9: Bilateral breathing	
6 × 75	Pull: free, with paddles and tube	On 1:30
6 × 75	Kick: free	On 1:45
	1st 25 of each 75 very fast	
150	Free	Swim-down

2,850 yards total

EMPHASIS: Building lung capacity and speed; conditioning through the use of drag

─────────────────────WORKOUT 115─────────────────────

Distance	Stroke	Time
150	Kick: free	Warm-up
150	Pull: free	
150	Free	
4 × 450	Free	# 1 on 7:00
		# 2 on 6:45
		# 3 on 6:30
450	Kick: free	
	Every 3rd 25, kick with head down	
	and breathe every 6 kicks.	
5 × 50	Head-out: free	On 1:10
450	Pull: free, with paddles	
	Breathe every 5 strokes.	
250	Free	Swim-down

3,650 yards total

EMPHASIS: Improving your oxygen-absorbing capability; leg and arm strengthening

─────────────────────WORKOUT 116─────────────────────

Distance	Stroke	Time
450	Free	Warm-up
	100: long strokes	
	100: ripple	
	100: Count strokes and keep	
	count consistent.	
	150: normal	
450	Free	
	Time yourself.	
450	Free, broken	Rest :20 after each 100.
	Beat preceding time by :20.	
450	Free, broken	Rest :10 after each 50.
	Beat preceding time by :10.	
18 × 25	Kick: free	On :30
100	Pull: free, with paddles and tube	Rest :20 after each
200	Lengthen stroke as distance	distance.
300	increases.	
18 × 25	Free	On :30
	Alternate 25 with head out and	
	25 with no breath.	
200	Free	Swim-down

3,500 yards total

EMPHASIS: Consistent pacing; breath control

─────────────────────**WORKOUT 117**─────────────────────

Distance	Stroke	Time
200	Free, long strokes	Warm-up
3,600 (144 lengths)	Free Alternate 10 lengths of bilateral breathing with 10 lengths of normal breathing.	
200	Free	Swim-down

4,000 yards total

EMPHASIS: Improving orientation to long periods of continuous swimming

─────────────────────**WORKOUT 118**─────────────────────

Distance	Stroke	Time
450	Free Breathe every 5 strokes.	Warm-up
8 × 200	Free Descend :05 on each 200. Last 200 = best time + :15.	On 3:00
450	Pull: free, with paddles and tube Breathe every 5 strokes.	
4 × 100	Kick: free Face in water. Breathe every 4 kicks.	On 2:00
200	Free	Swim-down

3,100 yards total

EMPHASIS: Holding pace; improving oxygen-absorbing capacity

─────────────────────WORKOUT 119─────────────────────

Distance	Stroke	Time
450	Free Alternate 50 kick and 50 pull and 50 swim.	Warm-up
900	Free Sprint 1st 300.	
4 × 150	Pull: free with paddles	On 2:30
3 × { 25 50 75 100	Free Lengthen stroke and decrease turnover rate as distance gets longer.	Rest :05. Rest :10. Rest :15. Rest :20
450	Kick: free Sprint every 2nd 50.	
200	Free	Swim-down

3,350 yards total

EMPHASIS: Starting fast and getting into your pace

─────────────────────WORKOUT 120─────────────────────

Distance	Stroke	Time
200	Free	Warm-up
150	Pull: free	
100	Kick: free	
50	Free	
6 × 200	Pull: free # 1–2: with pull buoy only # 3–4: with buoy and paddles # 5–6: with buoy, paddles, and tube	On 3:15
100s	Free Swim until you can't make interval. Then do 2 more on last interval made.	Best 100-yard time + 1:00 = 1st interval. Subtract :05 more on each subsequent interval.
6 × 75	Kick: free, broken	Rest :05 at 50 and kick with head down (no breathing) as far as possible on 3rd 25. On 1:30
450	Free, with fins	Time yourself.
200	Free	Swim-down

2,800 yards, plus 100s, total

EMPHASIS: Upper body conditioning; building strength against resistance; improving endurance

9

SWIMMING IN OPEN WATER

To me, the ultimate swimming experience is gliding along in the open water, with fingers of sunlight filtering their way up from the depths and a pool wall nowhere in sight—only the wide open spaces. I love the freedom and the feeling of being in with the elements that open water swimming affords, and I wonder why I haven't been indulging in such a treat for years. Unfortunately, except on the professional circuit, I'd never heard of any open water races, if they even existed. Now, on the other hand, open water races for experienced as well as novice competitive swimmers are plentiful.

But having an enjoyable open water experience means making the proper preparations. And preparing properly, as emphasized in preceeding chapters, begins with conditioning in the pool where you can use a pace clock and measure your distances accurately so that you exercise the discipline necessary to your training. It is still important, however, to spend time swimming in open water to get used to various sensations you may have when you race.

TECHNIQUES

Starting with the beginning of the race, the first occurrence you'll face is having that inviting deep blue or green expanse of

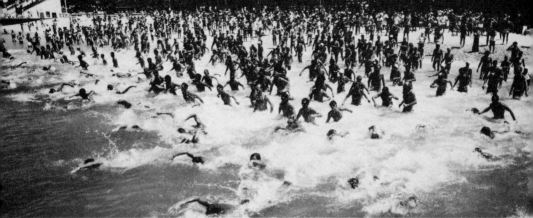

A crowd at the beginning of an open-water swim

water in front of you turn into a nightmare of thrashing arms and legs after the starting gun goes off. If you're not careful, your friendly feelings of being one with nature may turn to panic— particularly if you're trying to swim your way through this mass of humanity. In fact, one of the two greatest causes of panic in open water swimming is the insecurity that arises from the difficulty of finding free space to swim in.

Here are some points to consider when swimming among large numbers of people at the start of a race:

1. You can always wait before you take off from shore. If you are particularly frightened about the thrashing arms and legs of other swimmers, you can position yourself behind or off to the side of everyone else at the start, and if there are any marker buoys to be rounded, stay to the far side. After all, most contestants are looking for the fastest, shortest way and will therefore, scramble for a relatively small amount of space.

2. Other swimmers don't get in your way on purpose. Running into you slows them down as much as it does you, so don't feel angry or offended.

3. Water tends to cushion blows. Being kicked by another swimmer, although it may cause momentary loss of concentration, does not incapacitate you and causes only little, if any, pain.

4. You *can* swim with filled or poorly positioned goggles. If you wear goggles and they are knocked askew by another swimmer, either leave them alone or (with one hand) pull

them down around your neck until you are in open space and can roll over on your back and kick while readjusting them.

5. You can sprint out ahead of a crowd if your strength and endurance are good. Do this only if you are an experienced, well-conditioned swimmer who won't be exhausted by this technique.

6. The crowd usually thins quite rapidly. Whatever problems you may have concerning limited space will probably be short-lived.

The other major cause of panic is cold water, or perhaps I should say the anxiety caused by the first sensation of water that is colder than pool temperature (76–80 degrees Farenheit). You may experience a gasping sensation upon submersion the first few times you swim in the open water simply because you lack the confidence to handle yourself in water that, though not cold enough to affect you physiologically, is a new experience for you. This sensation can be overcome by relaxing your breathing and stroke as much as possible. It's not necessary to stop swimming, although you may want to swim with your head out until you stop gasping. Above all, don't panic! Also, realize now that the more times you can experience the colder temperature of open water before the race, the less likely it is that you'll be shaken up during the race. In addition, you may wish to immerse yourself a few minutes prior to the race or at least splash water on your face and arms.

Once you've been in the water a while and you're away from the crowd, you may get the feeling that everyone is ahead of you, or that you're all alone and can't see the bottom. Also, you may feel cold or warm spots or see debris floating in the water. Again, panic will only make things worse. Instead, try thinking about the same things you concentrate on when you're in the pool: proper stroke technique, complete exhalation, and the sensation of being in a different medium.

Staying on Course

Now let's discuss staying on course so you don't end up truly alone in the water. Following a course begins with choosing one or more conspicuous landmarks, such as a building, hill, or clump of

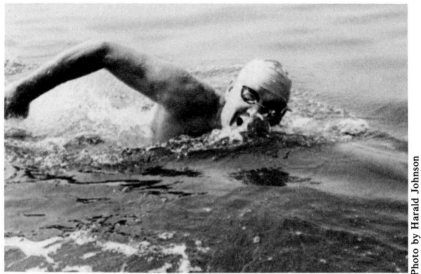

Photo by Harald Johnson

When following a course in open-water swimming, choose a landmark and limit raising your head to once every 8 or 10 strokes.

trees, that are in line with the marked course. The point is to find the way to your destination with the least possible alteration in your stroke and breathing. For example, I have on more than one occasion been swimming toward an orange buoy and lifted my head to look on three consecutive breaths just to make sure that what I saw ahead was indeed a marker and not somebody's orange-capped head. Had I selected an object that rose above the horizon, I'm sure one look would have been sufficient and I probably wouldn't have had to lift my head so high.

Lifting your head wastes both time and energy, but it is necessary to some degree when trying to keep your direction. Train yourself to limit raising your head to once every 8 or 10 strokes and to pick out reliable swimmers to follow in a race so that you can get away with looking even less.

Bear in mind that there may be instances when you deliberately want to aim off to the side of a course marker because of a current. Always study currents before a race and, if necessary, ask a race official about any known currents.

Waves may obscure your view somewhat and cause inconvenience but with a little extra effort and planning they need not be a problem. You may have to lift your head just a little higher to see, and you might want to learn to breathe on either your right or your left sides so that you can always be turning your face away from any on-coming waves. If you encounter waves coming toward you as you're going out in the beginning of a race, be sure to duck under them rather than trying to go through them. Also bear in mind that if nothing else, dealing with waves will be more tiring than swimming in smooth water and you may wish to roll over on your back at some point or points and simply rest a bit.

In any case, whatever techniques you use to increase your efficiency in open-water swimming, they will clearly be improved by practice during your training.

TRAINING IN THE OPEN WATER

Although you would be wise to do the majority of your training in the pool, certain techniques can best be practiced in the open water. Probably the most important result of training in the actual race environment is a feeling of confidence and control, which is a tremendous asset once the starting gun goes off.

Practice running out from shore through shallow water and submerging by diving headlong when the water is about mid-thigh deep. If the water is quite cold, you may want to do your first few strokes with your head up as you adjust to the temperature. Force yourself to breathe deeply these first few moments, and you'll avoid gasping. If the water remains shallow for a long distance, try doing several headlong dives in succession, pushing off with your feet from the bottom after each one. Learn to do this quickly, since you probably will (at least eventually) want to move out ahead of the crowd in order to be competitive.

Once you've settled into your pace, practice looking at land-marks on shore with as little alteration in your stroke and breath-ing as possible. And try to gain your bearing to the point where you can go pretty much in a straight line for at least eight to ten strokes without looking ahead. Also, work on getting comfortable in any turbulence you may find.

As far as actual conditioning in the open water, a water-proof watch (preferably a digital one that can easily be read) and a fixed distance between two or more points are your best tools. Get your time for the distance and repeat it several times on different days so that you can at least roughly compare your performances. Remember, however, that currents, wind, and temperature can all affect your times. Even the number of strokes you take per minute will be influenced by waves, but this is probably a more accurate indicator of your pace than just straight time. Practice with your watch and experience the feeling of swimming at a comforable "X" number of strokes per minute. Then try X + 10 strokes and X + 20 strokes. Keep doing this until you can fall into a particular cadence without having to look at your watch. Some swimmers I know keep pace by the use of songs or rhymes. For example, a given distance might be 100 "Row-Row-Row-Your-Boats" or 25 "America-the-Beautifuls." The point to remember is that if the number of strokes you take per minute remains consistent, so will your pace.

Swimming with a friend who goes at or near the same speed as you can also help you learn to pace. You may even want to practice *drafting* off one another, a technique of swimming directly behind another person (as close as you can without actually touching) for the purpose of conserving energy. This is a strategy often used in open water racing.

An exception to your normal pace will probably be at the beginning of the race, when you're sprinting to beat the crowd, so during your training swims, start out fast and then ease into your distance pace so you can get used to recovery from a sprint while still swimming.

Finally, spend some time swimming into shallow water and determining at what point to stand up and run the rest of the way in to shore—and probably a little way up the beach as well, since the finish line of most races is a few yards up from the shoreline. A safe guideline is to swim in to the point where your hands touch the bottom as you stroke. (I often get on my feet before that point if I'm close behind someone and I see that person up and running. No one's going to get the edge on me if I can help it, even if we're not in the same age group!)

SOME POINTS TO CONSIDER

Open water swimming can be an exhilarating, satisfying experience if you consider a few things in addition to your physiological preparation.

First, think about your own safety. Swim only when you feel you can handle the distance, temperature, altitude, weather, and other conditions along with your own physical and mental state. Be aware that you can release a cramp in your calf by turning your toes up toward your knees and stretching the muscle. For cramps in other areas such as your thigh or your hand, go into a floating position and use massage. Above all, in open water, *never swim alone*—no matter how well-trained you are. I suggest beginning with short swims in moderate temperatures as you're building your confidence. Furthermore, always do some form of warm-up before swimming hard. This may take the form of stretching or jogging on the beach if the water is uncomfortably cold (say 62 degrees or colder), but if you can tolerate it, get in the water for a little, easy swim to loosen up. I almost always go in at least waist-deep and splash water on my arms and face. Some precautions against cold include the following:

1. Wear a swim cap, or even two caps, which should be international orange in color for visibility. For maximum insulation, wear a thick rubber cap with an orange cap over it and pull both down over your ears.
2. Put lamb's wool in your ears. Use a dab of vaseline and make a ball with the wool before inserting in your ear.
3. Coat your skin with lanolin or petroleum jelly—particularly your underarms, neck, wrists, and the back of your knees where the veins are close to the skin. This is also a good precaution against chafing where some portions of your skin may rub against others.
4. Consuming even moderate amounts of alcohol within three days prior to an open water event will make you more sensitive to cold.

The question of whether or not to wear goggles is one you'll want to answer. Consider that while goggles will reduce eye irritation in very salty water and will probably also contribute a modicum of warmth, they will also hinder your vision above water and they may leak or be knocked out of position. So weigh the alternatives carefully. Personally, I go without goggles in all but the saltiest water.

All in all, with a little planning and some intelligent training, your open water swims may well be the most enjoyable swimming experiences you'll have.

10

TRAINING TIPS

The laws of fluid mechanics are such that certain motions in the water contribute to effective forward movement and others do the opposite regardless of the particular stroke. The following are some principles to consider in your quest for maximum efficiency with all strokes.

GENERAL PRINCIPLES OF EFFECTIVENESS IN THE WATER

1. Maximize resistance while pushing backwards. Probably the most important principle at work for you when you swim is that the only way your body moves forward is by your push against the water in the opposite direction. It's the old physics principle of "for every action there is an equal and opposite reaction." So each time you begin your pull of any stroke be sure your palms are facing your feet and make certain that you lead your pull with your hands, not your elbows (don't let your elbows drop), so that you make use of the largest possible surface area of your forearm. Developing ankle flexibility as well will increase the usable surface area of your feet.

2. Minimize resistance during your recovery. Just as it is important to maximize resistance when applying the leverage needed to move forward, it is essential to minimize any other kind of resistance. Therefore, to extend your arm or arms forward during the final portion of

your recovery or to perform an underwater recovery, let your hands slice through the water in the most streamlined fashion. Also, any bend in your knees during your kick should be kept to the minimum necessary for proper execution of the kick, since this causes the legs to drag.

3. Time your strokes so that during your arm recovery you have propulsion from your legs and during your leg recovery you have propulsion from your arms. You will thus avoid any "dead spots" in your stroke.

4. Release tension from all parts of your body. Allow your arms to relax on the recovery. Don't turn your palms to a pitch that causes strain, and don't press your fingers together. Be loose enough in the shoulders to allow body roll in freestyle and backstroke and loose enough in your ankles to get a good backwards push with your feet.

5. Exhale completely. If you inhale before exhaling completely you will take in less oxygen and therefore fatigue more quickly. Deep breaths are always preferable to shallow ones. Ineffective breathing is difficult for a coach or supervisor to spot, so you must rely on your own concentration, but the reward is ample. When I corrected my breathing during the 200 backstroke, my time instantly dropped 4 seconds!

6. Exhale underwater. No matter what stroke you're doing, a face-down position allows you the greatest freedom of movement as well as the most buoyancy. So keep the waterline at your hairline. If your head is too high, your feet will be too low; if your head is too low, it will be difficult to get into position to breathe.

7. When breathing, allow your head to move independently of your upper body. Lift or turn your head with your neck and return to a facedown position as soon as you take a quick breath.

8. Streamline your body whenever possible. When you glide, push off from the wall, or dive, make sure your arms and legs are both together and straight and that your head is down with your ears between your arms.

9. Push off from the wall while underwater. Make sure that you don't break the surface as you streamline off the wall, since this decreases your efficiency.

10. Stay low to the water on your turns. It's not necessary to push yourself up out of the water as you turn around, only to bring your feet around to the proper position for a good, hard push off the wall.

CHECKLISTS FOR PROPER EXECUTION OF EACH STROKE

Freestyle

UNDERWATER ARM PULL

1. Pull pattern is an elongated "S."
2. Elbow is bent up to 90 degrees.
3. Elbow is high.
4. Arm is extended for maximum distance per stroke.

Freestyle: bent elbow

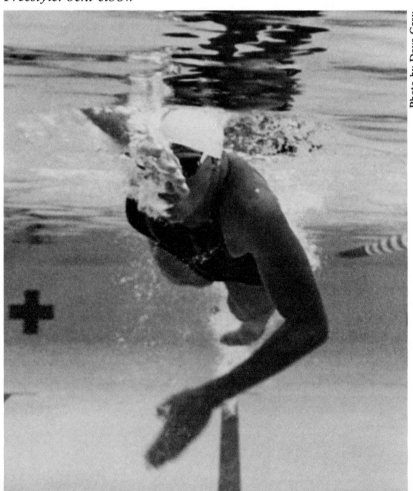

Photo by Dave Gray

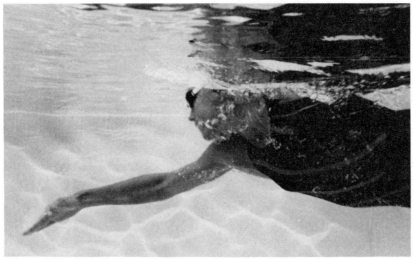

Photo by Dave Gray

Freestyle: arm extension

5. Hands accelerate through the stroke.
6. Body roll is present.
7. Hand entry is at a 45-degree angle.

ARM RECOVERY

1. Elbow is high.
2. Forearm is completely relaxed.
3. Hand enters water in front of shoulder.

KICK

1. Ankles are relaxed.
2. Knee bends slightly on downbeat.
3. Knee is straight on upbeat.
4. Only heels break the surface.
5. Kicks are small.

BODY POSITION AND BREATHING

1. Body is streamlined.
2. Water level is at the hairline.
3. Arms remain opposite one another.
4. Head is rolled, not lifted, to the side for inhalation.
5. Face is down for exhalation.
6. Exhalation is complete.

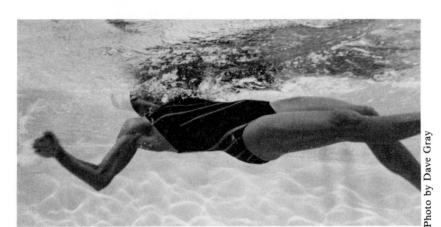

Backstroke: bent elbow

Backstroke

UNDERWATER ARM PULL

1. Pull pattern is an elongated "S."
2. Hand goes 12 to 18 inches (approximately 30 to 45 centimeters) deep before beginning the arm pull.
3. Hands accelerate through the stroke.
4. Body roll is present.
5. Elbow is bent up to 90 degrees.
6. Pull ends with palm facing down.
7. Hand enters little finger first.

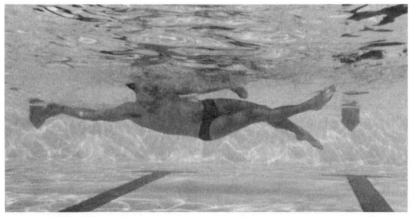

Backstroke: body roll and kick

ARM RECOVERY

1. Arm is straight.
2. Shoulder is lifted.
3. Hand enters water behind shoulder.

KICK

1. Ankles are relaxed.
2. Knee bends slightly on the upbeat.
3. Knee is straight on the downbeat.
4. Only toes break the surface.
5. Toes turn inward slightly.
6. Kicks are small.

BODY AND HEAD POSITION AND BREATHING

1. Body is streamlined.
2. Water level is in the middle of the head and just below the chin.
3. Head is positioned so that the line of vision forms a 45-degree angle with the surface and ears are in the water.
4. Arms remain opposite one another.
5. Breathing is in on one arm, out on the other.
6. Exhalation is complete.

Breaststroke

ARM STROKE

1. Simultaneous arm movements.
2. Arm pull pattern is heart-shaped.
3. One motion is used for pull and recovery.
4. Arms are extended in front of shoulders.
5. Elbows are high (just below the surface) during the pull.
6. Palms face backwards.
7. Hands pull back to chin level.
8. Palms face down during recovery.

KICK

1. Legs make the same motions at the same time.
2. Legs stay parallel to the surface.
3. At the starting point, legs are in a straight-back position with thighs together.

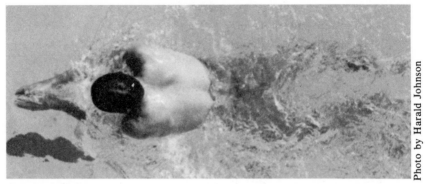

Proper breaststroke execution

4. Knees drop with thighs still together, feet relaxed.
5. Feet form right angles with shins and whip back in a half-circle motion, knees staying close together.
6. Hips rise at the end of the kick.
7. Feet do not break the surface.

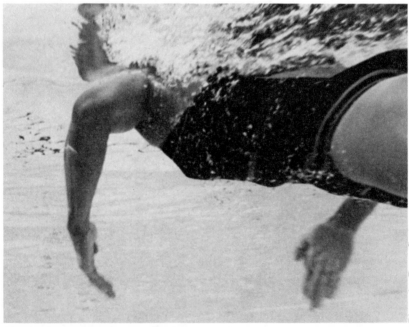

Breaststroke: high elbow

BODY POSITION AND BREATHING

1. Head breaks the surface at all times.
2. Heels are just below the surface.
3. Water level is at the hairline during exhalation.
4. Water level is just below the chin during inhalation.

TIMING

1. Arms begin their pull before legs begin their kick.
2. When hands reach chin level, knees begin to drop.
3. As knees begin to drop, head comes up for inhalation.
4. Before knees are fully dropped, hands come toward each other for recovery.
5. When knees are lowest, hands come forward.
6. Face submerges for exhalation as hands comes forward.

Butterfly

UNDERWATER ARM PULL

1. Pull pattern is an elongated "S."
2. Hands enter at 45-degree angle just outside shoulders.
3. Elbows are slightly raised at hand entry.
4. Arms are extended after hand entry.
5. Elbows are high throughout the pull.
6. Elbow is bent up to 90 degrees.
7. Hands are thrust backward and away from hips at the end of the pull.

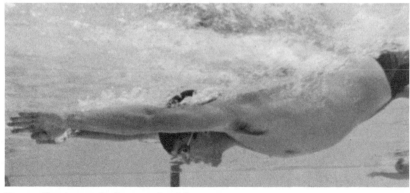

Butterfly: stretch forward with arms

Photo by Harald Johnson

ARM RECOVERY

1. Wrists relax when hands leave the water.
2. Hands swing forward just above the surface.
3. Elbows are straight or slightly raised.

KICK

1. Ankles are relaxed.
2. The kick is from the hips down.
3. Knee bends slightly on the downbeat.
4. Full knee extension causes hips to rise and break the surface.
5. Only heels break the surface.

BODY AND HEAD POSITION

1. Body bend is the key.
2. Head goes both lower and higher than in any other stroke.
3. Ears are between forearms on the stretch forward.
4. Chin is forward and just clears the surface during inhalation.

TIMING

1. Downbeat of the first kick comes when the arms enter the water in front.
2. Downbeat of the second kick comes as hands pass the hips.
3. Head reaches its highest point when feet are at the bottom of the second kick.
4. Head comes down as soon as possible after inhalation.
5. Breathing every other stroke provides optimal rhythm and body bend.

BENEFITS OF TRAINING DEVICES

Through the use of training devices, you can emphasize various aspects of your stroke to sharpen technique or build strength or both. Training devices also add variety and enjoyment to your regular swimming workouts.

Pull Buoy: A pull buoy is effective for isolating the arms for the purpose of working on stroke technique and for building arm strength. Such a flotation device keeps your lower body up in

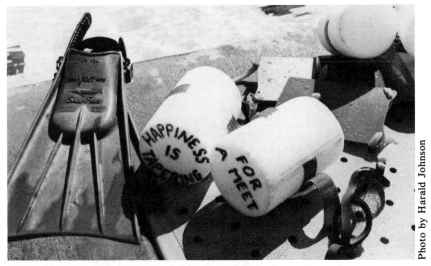

Swim fins, pull buoys, and hand paddles

swimming position without the necessity of kicking. A pull buoy is often used in conjunction with hand paddles and a tube to further overload the arms for the purpose of increasing the power of the arm stroke.

Hand Paddles: Hand paddles come in various sizes and shapes. Choose a size that extends ½ to 1 inch all the way around your palms. Also, some hand paddles have a lip extending away from your wrist so that if you attempt to lift your hand from the water before reaching the end of your stroke, you will encounter significant resistance, which will in turn encourage you to finish your stroke. Hand paddles are excellent for strengthening shoulder, chest, and back muscles because of the increased resistance of pulling a larger "hand" through the water. Your heart rate will be a little higher as well. But ease into your use of paddles and take care to train sparingly with them, since too much can cause soreness and even tendinitis.

Tube: You can further increase resistance during pulling by putting a small inner tube around your ankles to create additional drag. This will increase your heart rate and the level of stress on your arms, as using paddles does.

Kickboard: A kickboard serves as an aid in learning the proper mechanics of kicking and in building the leg strength necessary for

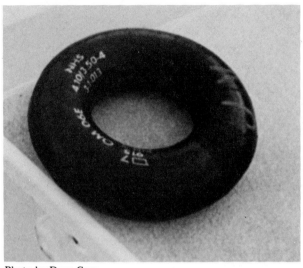

Tube for pulling

Photo by Dave Gray

efficient swimming. Through the use of a kickboard, the legs can be isolated from the rest of the stroke so that you can concentrate solely on kicking motions while maintaining body position. The same principle can be applied to building strength because, when propulsion comes solely from the legs, the heart must pump a tremendous volume of blood to the large muscles that are farthest from it, and this in turn creates a high heart rate as well as muscle stress. Leg strength, in turn, aids in maintaining good body

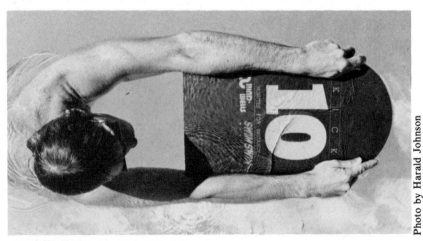

Kickboard

Photo by Harald Johnson

position, contributes to the power needed for fast sprints, and is crucial to a hard finish at the end of a race or a long swim.

Swim Fins: Swim fins help you develop ankle flexibility and are an invaluable aid to developing stroke technique because the added propulsion offers you additional balance and stability in your stroke. Fins are particularly useful for learning the butterfly because the extra power and undulation created by the kick allow you to get your arms up out of the water more easily. Also, when used while doing the backstroke, fins can be quite helpful for getting your hips and legs up into a good horizontal position. The shoe type of fins, which cover the whole foot except for the toes, stay on better and are more comfortable than the kind with the adjustable strap.

SPECIFICITY OF TRAINING

Any specific type of training that you do should always be preceeded by a solid base of general conditioning suitable to your level of ability. If you're starting back to swimming after a period of weeks or months away from the water, or if you've never swum for fitness or competition before, you'll definitely want to take the "I-have-plenty-of time" approach and begin moderately. If you're already at a good level of conditioning, your general base may be little different from that of a regular, more specific training program.

A solid base should consist of some basic work on stroke mechanics in addition to some general distance swimming to gain cardiovascular benefit, along with pulling and kicking to increase arm and leg conditioning. To determine the amount you want to do, look at your own level of conditioning and the level you want to attain and when you want to attain it. Review Chapter 2 on goal-setting.

Then, once you've assessed your direction and you've laid a general foundation of conditioning, you can begin to make your training specific to your goals. As previously mentioned, if you're going to specialize in distance events, you will want to emphasize long swims during your training more than short ones and if sprints are your focus, you should emphasize shorter swims.

But the question becomes: Where do you draw the line? I think it is as great a mistake to do *all* long freestyle training for distance freestyle events as to do none. Clearly, nothing prepares you better for an event than repeating it (or one very similar to it) over and over again beforehand.

However, I strongly believe that variety provides an invigorating change of pace that should not be ignored. For example, when I'm in training for open water swimming, I like to take two training sessions a week during which I emphasize strokes other than freestyle, even though I'm competing in freestyle only. I also think that varying the distances of repeat swims is of great value to maintaining motivation and interest.

You could, for instance, take a 500-yard freestyle distance and divide it in may ways (20 $\times$ 25 yards, 10 $\times$ 50 yards, 5 $\times$ 100 yards, 25-50-75-100-100-75-50-25 yards, 200-200-100 yards, or 200-150-100-50 yards). And on top of those variations, you could take short rest intervals (5–10 seconds) to emphasize endurance and consistent pace or long rest intervals (30 seconds or more) to emphasize speed. So there are a number of options available to you. It is hoped that, with a little forethought, you will be able to combine variety in your training with the specificity you need for top performance.

If it's truly top competitive performance you're seeking, you'll probably want to make your training still more specific than simulating the race events in practice. To do this, you'll want to arrange your training according to a three-part swimming "season" consisting of early-season, mid-season, and taper training. The purpose of these phases, when followed in sequence, is to help you achieve a physiological peak conducive to maximum performance at a predesignated time immediately following the taper period.

During early-season training (which is really nothing more than building an extensive solid base), the underlying goal is to lay the groundwork for the more strenuous phase of training to follow. Build a foundation of good stroke mechanics by spending some time doing one-arm swimming (right-arm stroking, then left-arm stroking) and isolating parts of your stroke with flotation devices so that you can do intensive work on parts of the stroke at a time and develop the psychology of constantly analyzing the efficiency of your movement. Also, spend some time perfecting your starts and turns and some long swims at a moderate pace to build the basic cardiovascular capacity necessary for higher-stress swimming.

Mid-season training is the most strenuous workout phase. Characteristic of this period, in comparison with earlier training, is swimming of a higher intensity, shorter rest intervals, and often greater total distance. Thus cardiovascular benefit during mid-season training is increased, since the heart rate is higher, does not drop as significantly, and remains high for longer periods. Your mid-season training should be closer to the maximum amount you can handle without excessive fatigue than it is in any other phase of your training. You must practice fast to be fast, and you must specialize at least to some degree in the stroke or strokes you wish to particularly excel in.

The taper phase is when the culmination of your dedication and strategy comes; the time when you allow your body to rest and come to its full strength; the time when you will swim the fastest and take the longest rest intervals, while spending the least time in the water. Characteristic of a taper workout are a thorough warm-up followed by a few short-fast swims at race speed, some dives and turns, and a swim-down. If you've trained hard, you need rest to put the icing on the cake, and you shouldn't be afraid to spend as little as 20–25 minutes per session in the pool the last few days before an important event.

While a swimming "season" serves to encourage a certain specificity of training, it is a long-term program, and the desired results can probably be attained only once or twice a year.

PUTTING IT ALL TOGETHER: SOME THOUGHTS TO REMEMBER

1. You don't have to be an expert, a super athlete, or even look good in a bathing suit to get started swimming. Do it now. You can get organized and set some goals for yourself after you get started.
2. Begin gradually using your heart rate as a guide. If you're just starting out and your swimming is fitness-oriented, stick to a target working heart rate of 60 percent of the difference between your resting and maximum heart rate over and above your resting heart rate. If you're well-conditioned and are interested in competition, train at up to 80 percent.
3. Pay attention to stroke technique and, if possible, have a specialist analyze your efficiency in the water.

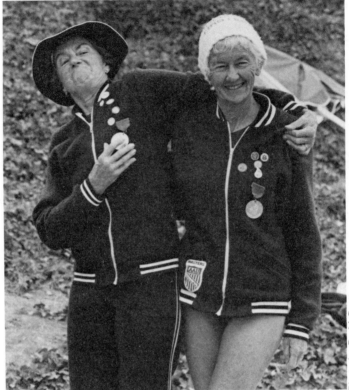

Photo by Budd Symes

Senior swimmers, proud of their achievements

4. Above all, swim regularly—at least three times a week for fitness, and more if it's competition you're interested in.
5. Keep your heart rate at a "working level" for at least 20 minutes per session to maintain a minimum level of fitness. Again, you'll want to do more if you want to compete.
6. Identify goals for yourself. And as you do so, never mind other people's goals. It's your own that will be appropriate for you and your schedule, and—most importantly—your own that will excite *you.*
7. Get yourself the proper equipment. Have a suit, cap, and goggles that you can live with comfortably. A pull buoy and kickboard will also be helpful for your training. If you want to do it all, throw in hand paddles, swim fins, and a tube as well.
8. Make your training specific for the kinds of events or distances you wish to excel in, but don't ignore the kind of variety in your training that keeps your interest fresh.

GLOSSARY

Abbreviations used in workouts:

Back = Backstroke
Breast = Breaststroke
Fly = Butterfly
Free = Freestyle
I.M. = Individual Medley

Bilateral: the term referring to breathing alternately on the right and left sides during freestyle.

Board: A board, or kickboard, is a nearly rectangular piece of buoyant material large enough to give support to the arms during kicking drills but small enough to handle easily during turns.

Broken: the situation resulting when a rest interval or intervals is inserted within a swim.

Catch-Up: the method of swimming freestyle in which each arm completes one whole stroke cycle, coming to rest in the forward position, before the other arm begins its cycle. In other words, the arms catch up with each other in front.

111

Descending: doing a series of swims of equal distance, each faster than the preceding swim.

Drafting: swimming directly behind another person, as close as possible without touching. This strategy conserves energy and is often used in open-water racing.

Eggbeater Kick: a breaststroke kick, but one leg at a time.

Individual Medley (I.M.): an event consisting of equal distances of butterfly, backstroke, breaststroke, and freestyle—in that order.

Interval Training: a type of conditioning consisting of periods of submaximal exercise alternating with controlled, short rest periods. Interval swimming can involve beginning each set at a fixed departure time, or getting a fixed amount of rest between each set, or interspersing occasional easily paced lengths between sets.

Kickboard: *See* Board.

Left-Arm Swimming: stroking with your left arm only, your right arm extended directly in front of you, using the freestyle stroke unless otherwise stated.

Long Strokes: a type of stroking used in freestyle and backstroke in which one arm stretches as far forward as possible while the other arm stretches fully to the rear in a slightly exaggerated fashion.

Mixed Strokes: doing the arm pull of one stroke while doing the kick of another stroke.

Negative Split: the situation resulting when the second half of a swim is faster than the first.

Paddles: plastic plates which come in various shapes and fit on the palms for the purpose of adding resistance and thereby building strength.

Progressive: the situation resulting when each length of a swim becomes increasingly faster than the preceding length.

Pull Buoy: a flotation device made of two Styrofoam cylinders fastened together and used for supporting the legs during pulling drills so that the arms are isolated.

Recovery: the portion of the stroke during which the arms or legs return to the position from which they begin propulsion.

Repeat: one swim in a series of swims of equal distance.

Right-Arm Swimming: stroking with your right arm only, your left arm extended directly in front of you, using the freestyle stroke unless otherwise stated.

Ripple: a stroke in which the fingertips touch the surface of the water during the entire recovery phase in freestyle, creating ripples on the surface.

Sprint Event: a swimming event of 100 yards or less.

Streamlining: the act of making the body as aquadynamic as possible by pointing the toes, straightening the elbows, keeping the head down, and in general creating as little resistance as possible.

Stroke: an arm cycle with either the right or the left arm, meaning that a complete arm stroke with both arms constitutes two strokes.

Tube: a small scooter-sized inner tube that wraps around the ankles to add resistance and build strength during pulling.

BIBLIOGRAPHY

Brems, Marianne. *101 Favorite Swimming Workouts*. San Mateo, California: Workouts, 1980.

———. *Swim for Fitness*. San Francisco: Chronicle Books, 1979.

DeVries, Herbert A. *Physiology of Exercise for Physical Education*. Philadelphia: W. B. Saunders Co., 1976.